SMALL ANIMAL ALLERGY:

A Practical Guide

SMALL ANIMAL ALLERGY:
A Practical Guide

Edward Baker, V.M.D.
Animal Skin and Allergy Clinic
Demarest, New Jersey

Lea & Febiger • Philadelphia • London • 1990

Lea & Febiger
200 Chester Field Parkway
Malvern, Pennsylvania   19355-9725
U.S.A.
(215) 251-2230
1-800-444-1785

Lea & Febiger (UK) Ltd.
145a Croydon Road
Beckenham, Kent BR3 3RB
U.K.

Library of Congress Cataloging-in-Publication Data

Baker, Edward, V.M.D.
    Small animal allergy : a practical guide / Edward Baker.
        p.   cm.
    Includes bibliographical references.
    ISBN 0-8121-1240-7
    1. Allergy in dogs.   2. Allergy in cats. 3. Veterinary allergy.
I. Title.
    [DNLM: 1. Animals, Domestic—immunology.   2. Hypersensitivity—
veterinary.   SF 910.H5 B167s]
    SF992.A44B35   1990
    636.7′089697—dc20
    DNLM/DLC
    for Library of Congress   90-5615
                                                                       CIP

Reprints of chapters may be purchased from Lea & Febiger in quantities of 100 or more.

PRINTED IN THE UNITED STATES OF AMERICA

Print number: 5   4   3   2   1

DEDICATION

This book is dedicated to my wife, Rosella, without whose encouragement and support this book would not have been written, to our daughters, Jane and Barbara, and our son-in-law, Roger, who are all talented writers in their own right, and to our granddaughter, Rachel, who is a great joy in our life.

PREFACE

I have always lived with allergies. As a child, I remember the severity with which my mother was afflicted with hay fever each fall. During my third year in veterinary school, I had my own first experience with allergy while currying a horse in the medicine ward, tearing and sneezing with each stroke of the brush. Diphenhydramine had just been introduced, and I remember how peacefully I slept at my desk by a sunny window, during a not-too-interesting lecture on the diseases of livestock. And finally, because my wife is also allergic, perhaps I have become more "sensitive" to the possibility of allergic disease and the variability of its clinical signs.

When I first entered practice in 1950, some segments of clinical medicine were still a complex mixture of ignorance, voodoo, and witchcraft. All seasonal skin diseases were due either to fleas or some combination of hot blood, thick blood, thin blood, too much protein in the diet, not enough protein in the diet, and other assorted equally "scientific causes."

It did not take long to recognize that the onset of many summer skin problems coincided with the onset of my mother's and other friends' seasonal allergy attacks. By the mid-1950s, I was experimenting with allergy skin tests on a limited basis, and within a year or two I had begun using immunotherapy for the treatment of seasonal dermatitis.

The concept of inhalant allergies was not accepted graciously in those days, especially by the academic community. In fact, I remember writing to a now prominent dermatologist/allergist, to suggest that inhalant allergy should be considered as one of the causes of skin disease, only to receive the reply that "allergy was an interesting curiosity in the dog, but would never amount to anything, clinically."

We were met with the same skepticism and, in some cases, derision, when I and a few others began talking about food allergy in dogs and cats. Acceptance came slowly, but there is no doubt about the regard in which food allergy is held today.

This book, then, is a labor of love—love for a field of medicine that has perplexed and fascinated me since I first stumbled into it some 35 years ago. It is also a vindication of a stubborn tenacity to pursue a concept, undaunted, in spite of occasional ridicule or being shoved out of the mainstream and beyond the pale of orthodoxy.

I have tried to transfer the information I have gathered over the years in a clear and practical manner, explaining what I do, how I do it, and why. Much of what follows is based on observation and personal experience. Some has also been extrapolated from human medicine, following many conversations with allergists and immunologists, combing the allergy journals, and attending innumerable allergy meetings and conferences. In recent years, as interest in animal allergy has grown, veterinary immunologists such as Drs. Ronald Schultz, Kevin Schultz, Richard Halliwell, Peter Eyre, and Ian Tizard have been gracious in sharing information, for which I will always be grateful.

Over the years, I sought answers to the questions that bothered me, and I now pass the information on. It is my sincere hope that the reader will find it a clinically useful text and one that will be referred to on a regular basis.

I thank Drs. Sandy Williams and Karen Feder for their comments in reviewing sections of the book. Thanks are also due to Mr. Peter Houck of Center Laboratories, Port

Washington, New York, for supplying much of the information on the relative significance and allergenicity of the various pollens and molds discussed in the chapter on aeroallergens.

I also thank my editors at Lea & Febiger for their confidence in this project and for their guidance during the writing and completion of this book.

Finally, I express my especial appreciation to Dr. Kevin Schultz of the Department of Pathobiology, School of Veterinary Medicine, Madison, Wisconsin, for giving so generously of his precious time in order to review this book. His perspectives and advice as both an immunologist and a clinician were invaluable and contributed in no small measure to the preparation of this text.

Demarest, New Jersey   Edward Baker

CONTENTS

Introduction

Considered little more than a clinical curiosity as recently as 20 years ago, allergy is now probably the "hottest" subject in the field of veterinary clinical medicine. Although formerly it was derided as lying somewhere between black magic and charlatanism, rarely is a meeting now held in which some aspect of allergic diseases is not on the program.

This change is hardly surprising because even the most conservative estimates suggest that at least 15% of the 55 million known dogs in the United States, and an unknown percentage of the feline population, suffer from allergic diseases. When converted into real numbers, this represents over 8 million potential canine patients alone. To this statistic must be added a large number of cats with skin, respiratory, and gastrointestinal problems, many of which will ultimately be shown to be allergic, as well as an increasing number of horses, cattle, and other species reported to have allergic reactions.

Even these numbers, however, do not truly explain the importance of allergic diseases to a clinical practice. In terms of *patients' visits*, allergic diseases can easily account for 50% or more of office practice, depending on time of year and geographic location. Even without absolute statistical evidence, allergic diseases potentially represent the third largest field of veterinary practice, following annual physical examinations/vaccinations and heartworm prevention.

The diagnosis and management of allergic diseases are neither obscure nor esoteric. Even though our current understanding of the pathophysiology of allergy and our knowledge of immunotherapy are imperfect at best, this should not be a deterrent to the successful management of the allergic patient. Over 70 years ago, with little or no knowledge of immunologic principles, physicians developed excellent diagnostic and management skills and offered welcome alternatives to the worthless nostrums available at that time.

As veterinarians today, we are in an enviable position, compared with that of these medical pioneers. Our diagnostic and treatment extracts are purer, better standardized, and more antigenically potent; new forms of allergenic extracts become available to us virtually as quickly as they become available to the physician; and because the pathobiology of allergic disease in man and the dog are almost identical, we can share observations while reaping the benefit of research in human medicine.

Allergy—What Is It?

The term *allergy* was coined by Von Pirquet[1] and means, literally, "altered reactivity." At the time, the normally functioning body, working at optimum capacity, was considered to be in a state of "ergy," a concept roughly derived from the Greek word meaning work. "Hyperergy" referred to a state of increased reactivity; "hypoergy," a state of decreased reactivity; and "anergy," a state in which an anticipated reaction did not occur. Because language is a dynamic process, only allergy and anergy have survived and are still in use, even though their meanings have changed.

It is interesting to note that allergy no longer means what it did to Von Pirquet. As originally conceived, the altered state was undefined—a change in any direction from the norm. Only with the passage of time and the inevitable refinement in concept and usage did allergy come to mean a state of increased or hyperreactivity.

HYPERSENSITIVITY AND SENSITIVITY

The terms *hypersensitivity* and *sensitivity* also are used in much the same way as allergy, referring to the reaction seen following exposure to an antigen or hapten as a result of a specific immune response to a prior exposure to the same agent.

Although allergy is not as descriptive a term as hypersensitivity and sensitivity, it is unlikely to be dropped soon from our diagnostic and descriptive terminology because it has become thoroughly ingrained in our language. Yet it is imprecise and often is used in a broad generic sense when other terminology would be more accurate or descriptive. As currently used, allergy exists when an individual reacts adversely to a substance that does not affect the bulk of the population. The reaction is mediated by the immune system and can range from mild to severe. Probably the best-known example in human beings is hay fever, in which up to 85% of the population can be exposed to ragweed pollen with no adverse effect, whereas the remaining 15% develop symptoms ranging in severity from mild coryza and rhinitis to asthma.

ATOPY

Atopy, on the other hand, was a specific syndrome to Coca when he first conceived and described it.[1] He did not consider it synonymous with allergy, but rather used it to describe certain forms of clinical hypersensitivity in man that were genetically determined and, most significantly, *"did not occur in lower animals."* As we now know, atopy does, indeed, occur in other species, particularly in the dog.

Allergy and atopy have become almost synonymous through common usage, especially in regard to inhalant allergies. Strictly speaking, however, all atopy fits under the canopy of allergy, although many allergic conditions, such as contact allergy and some forms of food allergy, are not atopic.

ALLERGEN AND ANTIGEN

An *allergen* is nothing more than an antigen, but with a narrower and more specific meaning. Whereas an *antigen* is any agent that either can stimulate an immune reaction or combine with a specific antibody, an allergen refers specifically to an antigen that stimulates an allergic response.

DESENSITIZATION, HYPOSENSITIZATION, AND IMMUNOTHERAPY

The terms *desensitization, hyposensitization,* and *immunotherapy* are frequently used interchangeably, although they do not necessarily mean the same thing. Desensitization would suggest that allergy injection therapy results in a total loss of sensitivity.

This would be unlikely in actual practice, and the term is therefore seldom used any longer. It was eventually replaced by hyposensitization because our current understanding of the events associated with injection therapy is that it actually only reduces the probability of a sensitivity reaction and a clinical response. The descriptive term in current general use is immunotherapy, which is another example of terminology changing with time. Although, classically, the term immunotherapy refers to passive protection achieved through use of hyperimmune serum or globulin, it has recently been applied to allergy injection therapy or, probably, to any biologic therapy, where the intent is to achieve a favorable clinical response by altering the immune system through the use of specific antigens or nonspecific immune modulators.

ATOPIC DERMATITIS

Atopic dermatitis is another term that was originally meant to apply only to humans and to specific forms of human allergic eczematous dermatitis. One reason, again, that "lower" animals were not included in the early definition was that they were not considered to suffer from true atopic allergic disease. In addition, the comparative aspects of skin disease were generally misinterpreted and misdiagnosed by the veterinary profession until recently, so both cause and diagnosis were usually ascribed to something other than allergy. Since those early days, both our understanding and our use of the term have changed. Now one may refer to atopic dermatitis in the dog or any other animal known to suffer from genetically determined, immunoglobulin (IgE) induced, allergic eczematous dermatitis.

Indeed, the three generally recognized forms of atopic dermatitis described in man can occur in the dog. Whereas the various syndromes seen in man can be conveniently grouped into broad general age categories, we are denied this luxury in animals. For example, atopic dermatitis in the infant and young child commonly involves the face, whereas in young adults, the antecubital areas and axillae are commonly affected. In more mature individuals, lesions are frequently found in the popliteal region and posterior thighs. These are the same regions in which lesions commonly occur in the dog, but they usually are concurrent and appear at any age.

A number of years ago, I spoke on food allergy in the cat at an international meeting of pediatric allergists. A group of my slides were of cats with some of the typical ulcerative lesions of the face so characteristic of food allergy. I vividly remember a midwestern allergist speaking to me later and saying how closely he could identify with my patients because so many of the young children that he treated for food allergy scratched their faces until they gouged out ulcerative lesions in the same places.

BLOCKING ANTIBODY

Blocking antibody is an antibody of the IgG class, produced when an allergen is introduced into the body through an abnormal route. For example, inhaled allergens normally produce IgE antibodies capable of causing an allergic reaction. Theoretically, the same allergen introduced subcutaneously during immunotherapy would produce a blocking antibody of the IgG class. Following successful immunotherapy, an allergen entering the body by a normal route would then encounter a circulating IgG-blocking antibody, combine with it, and be neutralized, thus preventing an allergic response. Although this was accepted dogma 10 to 15 years ago, we now know that this is too simplistic a view, and as we shall discuss later, apparently other things occur within the body and contribute to the reduction of sensitivity.

REFERENCE
1. Samter, M.: Excerpts From Classics in Allergy. Edited for the 25th Anniversary Committee of the American Academy of Allergy. Columbus, Ross Laboratories, 1969.

Immunology of Allergy

Allergy is an immune-mediated disorder involving antigens, antibodies, and complex biologic reactions, culminating in a host of clinical responses that can be distressing to both patient and owner. Allergy is not a single disease, but must be viewed in a generic sense, in that different types (such as inhalant, food, contact) involve different parts of the immune system and may initiate different clinical responses.

A detailed understanding of the immune system and its host/antigen relationships is not essential to diagnosis; however, the more one knows about these mechanisms, the better one is able to understand what is happening to the patient, how to diagnose and manage allergic disease, and what to do when the response to treatment is unsatisfactory.

Integral to this is a basic understanding of the four types of immune reactions, as classified by Gell and Coombs.[1] The actual sequence of events in each type of reaction complex, and only the most basic elements are described in this chapter. Specific reactions are discussed in more detail later under the appropriate subject headings.

TYPES OF IMMUNE REACTIONS

Atopic allergy is caused by a type I reaction, in which an antigen reacts with antigen-specific immunogobulin E (IgE) antibodies attached to mast cells or basophils. These antigen/antibody complexes in turn, initiate a series of complex biochemical reactions within the cells, culminating in the release of inflammatory mediators.

The type II, or cytotoxic, reaction involves IgG or IgM antibodies, which activate complement and/or certain cytotoxic cells, such as macrophages or neutrophils, which then directly attack and injure target cells.

In the type III (Arthus, serum sickness) reaction, IgG antibody forms circulating immune complexes with antigen. These complexes, in turn, activate complement, initiate the complement cascade, and cause tissue damage to target cells.

The type IV reaction involves activated lymphocytes, rather than antibody or complement. The inflammation is caused by inflammatory mediators released by these activated lymphocytes as they attack foreign matter, bacteria, or other antigenic cells in an attempt to isolate the offending antigen (Table 2–1 and Fig. 2–1).

CLASSIFICATION OF ALLERGY

The three broad general classifications of allergy are: (1) immediate, exemplified by allergic inhalant disease (AID); (2) contact, which is a delayed, type IV, cell-mediated reaction; and (3) food, which is generally immediate, but is occasionally associated with type III and IV immune reactions. Type II reactions have been reported, but are questionable. Food and contact allergies are discussed later as separate entities.

Allergy, in the form commonly seen in veterinary practice, is a type I reaction, based on the Gell and Coombs classification. The principal components of the allergic reaction are the antigen (allergen) and the IgE antibody. Mast cells, mediators, and target tissues may be the overt indicators of the clinical problem, but take away the antigen or the antibody, and allergy ceases to exist; one cannot proceed without the other.

ANTIGENS

Antigens are generally protein substances with a molecular mass of at least 10,000 daltons. They may also be combined with lipid molecules to form lipoproteins or with sugars to form glycoproteins. Antigens can be either complete or incomplete. Complete antigens are large enough and have the proper molecular configuration to evoke an immune re-

Table 2–1. Classification of Immune Response

	Reaction Type	Effector Mechanism
Type I	Immediate/anaphylactic	IgE
Type II	Cytotoxic	IgG, IgM, complement, cytotoxic cells
Type III	Immune-complex	IgG, complement
Type IV	Cell-mediated (delayed)	Activated lymphocytes

sponse without additional carriers or changes in their structure. Incomplete antigens, called haptens, are too small to stimulate an immune response without the addition of a carrier protein. This structural change is important in contact allergy, as is discussed later.

ANTIBODIES

All antibodies are not the same, nor are they homogeneous within their groups. The basic structure of each class of antigen may be the same, but subtle molecular differences, and differences in receptor sites, make them specific for a particular antigen.

Molecular Structure

The four classes of antibodies recognized in the dog to date are IgM, IgG, IgA, and IgE. Structurally, all are branched, Y-shaped molecules consisting of two long "heavy" chains and two shorter "light" chains of sequenced amino acids and sugar molecules. Antibody classes differ in their molecular weight and amino acid composition and in that some function as single antibody units, or mono-

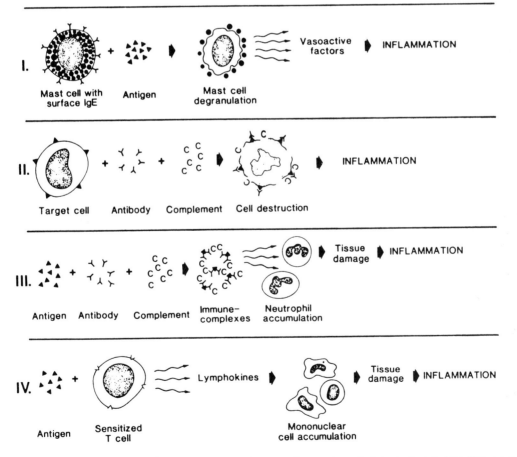

Fig. 2–1.   Types of immune reactions. (From Tizard, I.: Veterinary Immunology: An Introduction, 3rd Ed. Philadelphia, W.B. Saunders, 1987, p. 274.)

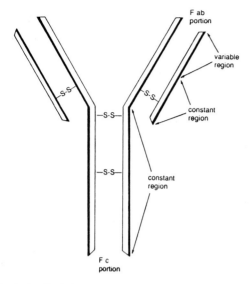

Fig. 2–2. Basic immunoglobulin structure (IgG, IgA, and IgE). IgG, IgE, and circulating IgA are monomers, whereas secretory IgA is a dimer and IgM is a pentamer. (From Baker, E.: Allergic reactions. *In* Canine Medicine, 4th Ed. Vol. 1. Edited by E.J. Catcott. Santa Barbara, CA, American Veterinary Publications, 1979.)

mers, whereas others are joined together into compound antibodies, or polymers (Fig. 2–2).

IgG and IgE are monomers, as is IgA while in the circulation, where it is apparently relatively inactive. IgA becomes activated when it is secreted through the mucosa into the lumen of the gut, respiratory tract, or other mucosal tissue. There it picks up a protein molecule called the "secretory piece," which then joins two IgA monomers into a dimer. IgM, on the other hand, is a pentamer, consisting of five antibody molecules linked together at the stem of the Y.

Functional Development

From a developmental standpoint, it would seem that IgM is the oldest or most primitive antibody class and the first to be mobilized against infection. IgM is soon replaced by IgG antibodies and gradually decreases as the concentration of IgG antibodies increases, leaving IgG as the principal antibody mobilized to fight infection after infection has entered the body. Because IgA is found on all mucosal surfaces, its principal role is to be on "surveillance patrol" at the portals of entry into the body, where it is prepared to intercept and destroy harmful antigens and infectious agents before they can enter the body and become established.

IgE has only been identified within the past 20 years as the antibody responsible for the type I reaction. In the older literature, before IgE was identified, it is referred to in several ways, such as reagin, reaginic antibody, and skin-sensitizing antibody. Although these terms are only of historical importance today, they can sometimes be confusing, especially to those who have entered the medical or veterinary profession since that time. Only skin-sensitizing antibody is still used occasionally.

Teleologically, the principal function of IgE apparently was to protect the individual from the ravages of helminth infections. Consequently, it seems apparent that any individual not suffering from an immune defect can produce this antibody. The puzzle facing allergists and immunologists is why this protective antibody evolved to be also disease producing for a limited segment of the population.

Genetic Considerations

Why 15 to 20% of the population should develop IgE antibodies capable of eliciting an allergic response is not clear. Immunogenetics play an important role in that although IgE can potentially reach a high concentration in any individual infected with migrating helminth larvae, the production of allergen-specific IgE depends on the individual's being genetically programmed to develop it. What also is not totally clear, in spite of our extensive knowledge of antibody production and immune-mediated inflammation, are the actual events that stimulate the immune system to produce IgE, rather than not to respond, and the cascade of events leading to the ultimate pathobiologic response. In other words, are these random events with allergens accidentally combining with antibodies, or are they somehow directed toward their specific antibodies?

Antigen Processing and the Immune Response

What is known can be summarized, so it is at least possible to have a basic understanding of these complex biologic and bio-chemical actions and reactions. Certain antigens, such as pollen grains and mold spores, apparently have a much greater ability to stimulate IgE production than do other foreign proteins. Such an allergen enters the body by crossing the natural body barriers of skin or mucous membranes. In the skin, it may contact a dendritic Langerhans cell, which then "processes" the antigen so it can stimulate an immune response. For those antigens passing through the mucosa, in order to develop an IgE antibody they must come in contact with a specialized macrophage, which instead of destroying the antigen, "processes" it for antibody stimulation. Regardless of route, the processed antigen is ultimately "presented" to a B lymphocyte, which, through the additional influence of "helper" T lymphocytes, is stimulated to produce large amounts of antigen-specific antibody. Clones, or families, of such lymphocytes are established and are capable of producing more antibody with each additional exposure.

Suppressor T lymphocytes also play a significant role in regulating the production of IgE antibody. As IgE levels increase, suppressor cells are activated and decrease or terminate IgE production. Perhaps the key to the induction of allergy lies within a defect in these suppressor cells that renders them incapable of regulating IgE and permits excessive amounts of antigen-specific antibody to develop.

Antibody molecules then circulate until they attach to special receptors sites on the cell membrane of the mast cell or basophil. Attachment is at the straight end of the Y-shaped antibody, the Fc fragment, so called because it becomes crystallized when the molecule is fractionated. The Fc fragment contains the antigenic determinants of the antibody molecule that enable it to attach to the receptor sites on the cell membrane.

At the end of each of the two arms of the Y-shaped antibody is the Fab fragment, referring to Antigen-Binding or AntiBody-active fragment. Unlike the straight tail of the Y, called the constant region, which remains identical from molecule to molecule, the Fab region is variable, allowing it to change shape to conform and bind to a vast number of antigens. Each antigen-binding site is specific for only one type of antigen, or one that is closely related antigenically. Allergens that get past the macrophages or Langerhans cells may ultimately attach to the combining site of the antibody and thereby may set off the chain of events that ultimately leads to an allergic reaction.

Fortunately, an antigen becoming attached to the antibody receptor site on just one antibody is not enough to initiate mast cell de-

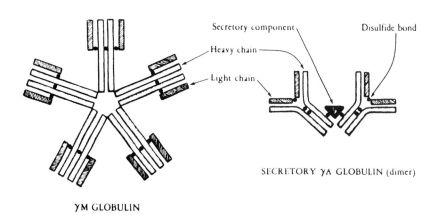

Fig. 2–3. Models of γM globulin, in its usual pentameric form, and secretory γA globulin, which is shown attached to a secretory component. Note the absence of the light-heavy interchain bonds in the γA globulin. The predominant γA globulin in secretions is of the γA2 subclass, which lacks such bonds. (From Bellanti, J.A.: Immunology. Philadelphia, W.B. Saunders, 1971, p. 105.)

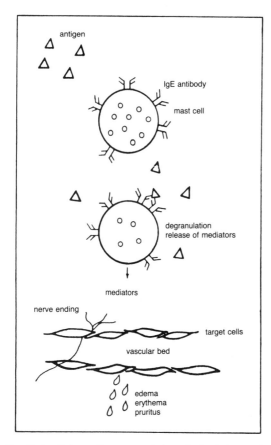

Fig. 2–4. Schematic representation of circulating antigens bridging two molecules of IgE attached to a mast cell. Subsequent biochemical reactions result in degranulation of the mast cell and release of allergy mediators. These mediators attach to receptor sites on target cells and thereby cause edema, erythema, and pruritus. (From Baker, E.: Allergic reactions. *In* Canine Medicine, 4th Ed. Vol. 1. Edited by E.J. Catcott. Santa Barbara, CA, American Veterinary Publications, 1979, p. 258.)

granulation and mediator release. To set the sequence of events in motion, the antigen must attach to, and bridge receptor sites on, two adjacent IgE molecules. Because attachment of the antibody to the mast cell membrane is a random event, antibodies may or may not attach to adjacent cell membrane receptor sites, and those that do may not necessarily have receptor sites for the same antigen (Figs. 2–3 and 2–4).

Degranulation and Mediator Release

Once the antibodies have been bridged, however, the chain reaction that has started must continue to its inexorable conclusion, unless specific preventive medications have been given or other measures have been taken to moderate the effect. Events within the mast cell occur rapidly. The mast cell granules are mobilized and migrate to the cell wall, with which they first fuse before being extruded through the cell wall and released.

When mast cell granules have been released into the surrounding tissue, extracellular fluid in some way initiates the release of vasoactive substances from the granules, leading ultimately to vasodilation, edema, smooth muscle constriction, inflammation, and pruritus. The principal mediators of significance in the dog and cat, whether released by the granules or synthesized from granule precursors, include histamine, leukotrienes, kinins, prostaglandins, heparin, platelet-activating factor, and eosinophil chemotactic factor.

The aim of treatment, then, as we shall see, is to block or alter the immune response, thus reducing the severity of the allergic attack or preventing it altogether. Such treatment can be directed toward several points. These include preventing the allergen from entering the body (much easier with foods or other ingestants than with inhalants); blocking the allergen from binding with IgE antibodies; finding some way to "turn on" a suppressed or "turned-off" suppressor T-lymphocyte system, and "stabilizing" mast cells or basophils, thus preventing mediator release. Much research is also devoted to the pharmacologic regulation of the mediators of immune inflammation, using antihistamines, antiprostaglandins, antiserotonin compounds, mast-cell stabilizing compounds, and nonspecific pharmacologic compounds.

The research community is optimistic that safe new medications, capable of controlling most allergic manifestations are on the immediate horizon. Until then, allergen identification by skin testing followed by immunotherapy offers the greatest hope of blocking antigen/antibody binding and inflammatory mediator release.

REFERENCE

1. Wright, R., and Robertson, D.: Immunologically mediated damage. *In* Food Allergy and Intolerance. Edited by J. Brostoff and S. Challacombe. London, Bailliere Tindall, 1987.

3 ‖ *History*

Probably the most tiresome phrase in clinical medicine is the basic truth, "there is no substitute for a good history." Yet nowhere in medicine can this be stressed more than in allergy and dermatology. A well-planned medical history, carefully taken, often gives you the diagnosis before the patient is even placed on the examination table.

The medical-history questionnaire has been designed as an all-purpose form (Fig. 3–1). The reasons for inclusion of specific questions are discussed; however, these are neither exhaustive nor necessarily significant for every practice. Therefore, the form can be easily modified and questions added or deleted to satisfy the needs of the individual clinician. The intent of the medical history is to aid in determining not only the type of allergy, but also whether an allergy even exists in a particular patient.

BACKGROUND HISTORY

Many allergic animals develop vague clinical signs early in life that often either go unnoticed or are considered insignificant by the client or the attending veterinarian. These signs become progressively more severe until the client suddenly realizes that the animal has a real problem. If the patient's early medical history is unknown because of late adoption or a change of owners, every effort should be made to try to contact the original owner and veterinarian to obtain this information.

The animal's original geographic area can provide important diagnostic clues because certain specific diseases are more prevalent in one area of the country than in others. For example, fungal infections affecting the skin or respiratory tract, such as histoplasmosis, cryptococcosis, or blastomycosis, are common in the Midwest, but rare in the Northeast. In addition, a pruritic puppy coming from a large puppy farm or poorly run pet shop or kennel is more likely to have mange than allergy.

The age of onset is important in allergy. When one has ruled out ectoparasites, the most common cause of pruritus beginning before the first birthday, particularly in animals under 6 months of age, is allergy, and the most common cause of allergy at this age is food. This situation gradually changes, so inhalant allergens become the most common cause in animals whose allergies first develop when they are around 18 months old. These are not absolutes, of course, and food and inhalant allergies are often concurrent, but they are good rules of thumb and serve as basic diagnostic guidelines.

SEASONALITY

Seasonal problems are invariably a result of seasonally prevalent inhalant allergens. By knowing the time of year clinical signs begin and end, the allergens commonly prevalent in the area, and their time of pollination or sporulation, one can pinpoint the most probable groups of inhalants responsible for the problem.

Nonseasonal problems, on the other hand, may be caused by inhalants, food, or both, and the diagnostic workup must be directed toward any of these possibilities. If nonseasonal allergies regularly worsen at certain times of the year, this would suggest that, regardless of cause, a seasonal inhalant allergen aggravates the condition during that time.

Clinical signs worsening at night suggest mold sensitivity, whereas problems worsening during the morning or midday suggest pollens. When clinical signs worsen in a specific location, such as indoors or out, at home or away, the patient is probably exposed to allergens either unique to that specific location or in an unusually high concentration.

HISTORY

Owner's name _____ Date _____

Address _____ Phone _____

Breed _____ Sex _____ Name _____ Age _____ Aged obtained _____

Obtained from: _____ Kennel _____ Pet shop _____ Breeder _____ Shelter _____ Private family

Which state _____ Has dog ever been out of local area?_____ State _____

If yes, explain _____

When were symptoms first seen? Age _____ Month _____ Year _____

Symptoms seasonal _____ Nonseasonal _____

If seasonal, in spring _____ Summer _____ Fall _____ Winter _____

If not seasonal, do symptoms get worse in any particular season? _____

Describe _____

Symptoms worse at night _____ Morning _____ At home _____ Away _____ Indoors _____

Outdoors _____ If indoors, any particular area _____

Other pets in house _____ Pets allowed on beds or furniture? _____

Type of heat: Hot air _____ Hot water _____ Steam _____ Air conditioning _____

Central _____ Window _____ Carpeting in home (type) _____

Type of bed pet sleeps on _____

If cushion, mattress or pillow used, what is it stuffed with?_____

Describe outdoor environment (lawn, wooded area) in which pet will run or play. Also describe types and variety of shrubs, grass, and weeds in environment _____

Are many potted plants kept in house? _____

Diet: Canned _____ Meal _____ Soft: moist _____ Dry _____ Kibble _____ Table food _____

Mixed table and prepared _____ Percentage of each _____

Does exposure to, contact with, or eating any of the following cause problems?

Cold _____ Dampness _____ Tobacco smoke _____ Wool _____ Dust _____ Perfume, after shave lotion, or cosmetics _____ Specific foods _____ Drugs _____ Other _____

Describe reaction _____

Allergic manifestations: Scratching _____ Running nose _____ Sneezing_____ Hives_____

Wheeze _____ Cough _____ Foot licking _____ Face rubbing _____ Diarrhea _____

Vomiting_____ Other_____

Describe _____

Any unusual activity just before onset of symptoms _____

Is pet nervous or easily upset emotionally? _____

Describe _____

Previous illness or infection _____

Was there a change in environment shortly before onset of symptoms?

Yes _____ No _____ If yes, explain _____

Is house New _____ Old _____ Dry _____ Damp _____ Any new furnishings in house just before problem started _____ If yes, explain _____

Has there been any major landscaping or other work done on the lawn or shrubs? Yes _____ No _____ If yes, explain _____

Are deodorants or fresheners used on carpet? Yes _____ No _____

If so, which _____

Was pet bathed, groomed, boarded or in a different environment before problem started? _____

Describe _____

If spayed, did condition start or worsen shortly after surgery? Yes _____ No _____

If unspayed, are heat cycles regular? Yes _____ No _____

  Does condition worsen when pet comes into heat? Yes _____ No _____

  If false pregnancy occurs, does condition worsen? Yes _____ No _____

  When in heat, is pet normally attractive to males? Yes _____ No _____

  When in heat, is pet normally interested in males? Yes _____ No _____

If male, is he normally interested in females in heat? Yes _____ No _____

Does condition worsen when stimulated by females in heat? Yes _____ No _____

If castrated male, did condition begin or worsen after surgery? Yes _____ No _____

Are medications currently being used? Yes _____ No _____

If so, what are they? _____

Do you think they help? _____

Explain _____

Have family members developed skin problems SINCE the pet's skin problem began? Yes _____ No _____

  Explain _____

Describe in your own words the problem for which the pet is being examined today _____

Describe any observations not already covered that you think would be of value _____

Fig. 3–1. Medical-history questionnaire.

OTHER ANIMALS

Determine whether other pets live in the house and whether they are also affected. If so, suspect a communicable problem, particularly fleas or mange, rather than allergy. It is unusual, although certainly not impossible, for two or more pets in the same household suddenly to become allergic at the same time.

ENVIRONMENTAL FACTORS

Find out whether the pet is allowed on the furniture, where it sleeps, and whether it has a bed of its own. In addition, try to determine the types of stuffings used in the bed and furniture, as well as the types of carpeting the pet may lie on. Cedar shavings in dog beds and kapok- or feather-stuffed pillows are common causes of allergy.

Carpets of wool, other natural fibers, and pattern-dyed synthetics, along with felt or other nonsynthetic padding, are more likely to produce allergy than synthetic carpets with foam rubber or synthetic padding. This does not mean that foam rubber is innocuous; contrary to popular belief, it supports heavy mold growth, especially as it ages.

Although synthetic carpeting is not usually allergenic, the clipped ends of the nap can be sharp and may occasionally irritate an animal's foot pads or hairless portions of the lower abdomen. In addition, even synthetic carpeting may have jute or other plant fibers incorporated into the backing, and these are often allergenic. Further, even though the synthetic fibers may not be allergenic, the dyes applied to them occasionally cause a contact allergic dermatitis.

Any type of heating system can set up convection currents that can aggravate allergies, but hot-air heat is probably the most serious offender because it forces out dust and mold spores and circulates them in the environment. This situation is particularly important when heating systems are first turned on in the fall, when particles have accumulated in the ducts for a long time.

The same is true of central air conditioners. Therefore, high-quality filters must be installed in the system, and the filters must be cleaned or serviced regularly.

The outdoor environment is probably the most important factor in inhalant allergy. Even though mold spores and pollens can blow for miles, initiating an allergic attack far from their point of origin, the clinical problem will be much worse if the immediate environment is heavily wooded, planted with shrubbery, or overgrown with weeds.

Shrubbery beds support heavy concentrations of mold growth and promote excessive exposure of mold-sensitive pets living in homes landscaped with luxuriant shrubbery. When these pets are allowed to dig in the shrubbery beds, exposure is further increased as masses of mold spores are stirred up. The same is true for house plants. Pots and soil are virtual mold factories that can aggravate an already sensitive patient, especially in a closed environment or an environment in which particles are actively distributed throughout the house by heating or cooling fans.

FOOD

One must take a dietary history to separate food from inhalant allergies. Many pet foods, especially some of the soft moist, heavily dyed varieties, have been implicated in food allergy and should be identified in the patient's history. Because prepared foods are such complex mixtures of meat and cereal "meals," individual food items, flavors, colors, and preservatives, it is difficult to determine just which ingredients are the offenders. Fresh table foods can also cause allergy, but because mixtures of individual foods are usually fed, it is generally easier to isolate and to identify them. Food allergy is discussed in more detail in Chapter 13.

CLIMATIC FACTORS

Cold temperatures are an uncommon cause of urticaria and mediator release. I have seen one dog that was so temperature sensitive that merely lying on the cold examining table was sufficient to cause hives and pruritus.

Damp, humid areas must be avoided because these serve as an excellent breeding environment for molds.

FUMES AND ODORS

Fumes and odors are actually suspended fine particulate matter and, as such, can be either respiratory irritants or true allergens. Among the most common offenders are tobacco smoke, perfume, after-shave lotions, and cosmetics. To illustrate the importance of tobacco smoke in sensitive animals, I recently saw a patient that was undergoing immunotherapy for a number of positive allergens, including tobacco. The animal was doing well until the family had a large party attended by heavy smokers. As the evening wore on and smoke filled the rooms, the dog became progressively more pruritic and the skin more inflamed. The condition did not improve until the dog was finally isolated in a well-ventilated area away from the smokers.

The other items mentioned are self-evident and are not intended to constitute a complete list. Rather, they should help to direct both the veterinarian and the client to thinking about things that may possibly incite a clinical reaction.

CLINICAL REACTIONS

The type of reaction evoked, as well as the allergic manifestation, helps to direct one's thinking to a specific organ system and the most probable type of allergen. Localized dermatitis on the thin-coated or hairless parts of the body suggests a contact allergy. Respiratory signs suggest an inhalant allergy, although food can cause asthma; generalized pruritus, face rubbing, and foot licking can result from either inhalant or food allergy. Gastrointestinal signs, hives, and angioedema are usually caused by foods, although drugs also occasionally cause such reactions. Nonetheless, there are no absolutes and these are only guidelines; any allergen can cause any type of clinical manifestation in any given patient.

CONTRIBUTING MEDICAL HISTORY

If allergic attacks are intermittent, with or without a specific pattern, it is important to try to pinpoint any specific or recurrent activity before the onset of an attack. High-spirited racing or other activity causing overheating may release cholinergic mediators, causing pruritus. A rare condition has also been described in man in which exercise after eating has produced anaphylaxis. The

mechanism responsible for the reaction has not been clarified, but clinical signs may include hypotension, asthma, angioedema, urticaria, and generalized anaphylaxis. Pizza parties, placement in a room or environment that is unusual for the patient, exposure to rarely used toys or pillows, and confinement in a kennel, dusty attic, or damp cellar are all potential sources of allergens and resultant reactions.

Nervous pets or those that are easily emotionally upset are potential neurotic scratchers. Previous illness, such as liver disease with wasting or jaundice, can lead to skin changes and alopecia, with or without pruritus. Some infections, especially those caused by viruses that are trophic for ectodermal tissue, can lead to hair loss, pruritus, and skin changes that are usually transient. When canine distemper was more common, dogs were sometimes presented for treatment with cornified foot pads, hyperkeratotic patches, and patchy or diffuse hair loss as part of the disease syndrome.

HOUSEHOLD FACTORS

Obtaining information about the house in which the pet lives can be invaluable. New houses frequently have remnants of sawdust and construction dusts that are allergenic and, although not obvious, can remain in the environment for long periods of time. Old houses, on the other hand, are bountiful sources of dust and mold. Dry homes generally cause the least number of problems, whereas damp homes generate masses of mold spores. New furnishings can also contain dusts, fabric particles, or dyes that can act either as irritants or allergens. Rug dry cleaning powders are often a source of severe persistent pruritus in some dogs. Molds released while working the soil during landscaping are a potentially severe problem for some dogs, as are the sawdust and construction dusts generated by building materials during remodeling and new construction.

An often overlooked problem during December and January is the Christmas tree; many dogs are sensitive to the molds and resins commonly associated with these trees.

Bathing can dry the coat, whereas harsh soaps or detergents can act as irritants.

Grooming powders or conditioners can also be either irritants or allergens.

Thus, as one begins to understand the patient's daily life and environment, the pattern that often develops helps to point one toward the most probable diagnosis.

HORMONAL INFLUENCES AND MEDICATION

Intact dogs sometimes have skin problems that develop or become exacerbated during estrus or pseudocyesis. In the male, this situation occasionally occurs when neighborhood females are in estrus. Females may develop erythema of the ventrum with inflamed and enlarged nipples, accompanied by severe pruritus. Males develop generalized pruritus, a more diffuse erythema, and an eczematous reaction.

Ovariohysterectomy and castration are curative. Whether this reaction is allergic or is caused by some other mechanism is uncertain. Intradermal skin tests using estrogens or progesterone have been used diagnostically by some allergists, although I know of no direct evidence to prove the validity of the test. The test injection is placed deeper than standard skin tests and may take up to 72 hours to react; a local inflammatory reaction may then be seen.

Medications that the patient is or has been receiving can affect the diagnosis and diagnostic/treatment plan. For example, certain medications, such as cephalosporins, neomycin, and sulfonamides have caused drug eruptions that can mimic allergy and other skin disorders. Other drugs, such as corticosteroids and antibiotics, can temporarily improve the condition or may change the typical characteristics of the lesion. Furthermore, if the patient was receiving corticosteroids, antihistamines, or phenothiazine-based tranquilizers, either during or shortly before allergy skin testing, these drugs could seriously diminish reactions and affect the test results.

COMMUNICABILITY

The patient's owner should be questioned about whether lesions have developed in family members or in any other person in close contact with the pet since the problem began. If so, one must then rule out any possibility of a communicable disease. If the affected individual has been to a physician, try to find out the diagnosis and whether it is consistent with the diagnosis of the pet's condition.

PERCEPTUAL CONSIDERATIONS

Asking the owner to describe why the pet is brought in for examination is always interesting because it gives one insights into how the owner thinks and the medical problems that worry him most. Clients often see things differently than we do, and conditions that have a high priority rating on our problem list may be of little or no concern to the owner. I have often had patients referred to me for a specific problem. Yet when I ask the owners what the problem is, they either do not know or have a totally different perception of why they brought in their pet.

The medical history form shown in Figure 3–1 is not meant to be complete and unchangeable for every practice, but rather it is designed as a framework on which to build. Veterinarians can use it as it is, can reject aspects unimportant to them, and can add questions important to their practice area. Above all, use a history report form. It can be completed by the client in the waiting room, or the questions can be asked by an assistant during a preexamination conference. As mentioned at the outset, a well-conceived and thoroughly executed medical history often suggests the diagnosis before it is ever confirmed on the examination table. Most important, even if it is not necessarily diagnostic, it will most certainly keep you on track and help to prevent you from overlooking significant information without which the final diagnosis might not be made.

Physical Examination and Laboratory Data Base

The three tenets that I consider basic to the evaluation and diagnosis of itching skin disease are as follows:

1. All that itches is not allergy.
2. All that is allergic does not itch, such as gastrointestinal and respiratory allergy.
3. A diagnosis of allergy is not justified until one has ruled out all other possible diagnoses.

Therefore, the physical examination must be complete and thorough. To minimize the possibility of distraction or of overlooking important details, it is best to establish a consistent pattern, or routine, of examination, following the same procedure each time. Use of an examination flow chart, such as illustrated in Figure 4–1, can help one to perform a consistently thorough examination.

GENERAL OBSERVATIONS

Before placing the patient on the table, observe the animal from a few feet away, to get an overall impression of the general appearance of the coat, conformation, attitude, and thriftiness. In particular, look for frequency and intensity of scratching, first while in the waiting room and later in the examination room. Most animals, when presented, are too nervous, excited, or curious to think about scratching. Therefore, if scratching is seen, it is more significant than pruritus that occurs only at home or while in a familiar environment.

Although the amount of scratching in the office is not an absolutely reliable diagnostic indicator, one may draw some preliminary general conclusions, which must then be confirmed or ruled out by further examination. For example, if a skin problem is not accompanied by pruritus, or if pruritus is minimal and the patient is easily distracted, an underlying or contributing metabolic dis-

ease will be high on the "rule out" list. If the patient scratches occasionally, with variable intensity, allergy will be the prime diagnostic probability. Intense and frequent pruritus could be due to allergy, but sarcoptic mange, fleas, and other ectoparasites are more likely to be highly pruritogenic and must be ruled out first.

Look for thinning of the coat, hair loss, and alopecia, and observe in particular whether it is randomly scattered or symmetric. Hair-loss patterns are not absolutes either, but they do provide clues to the directions one should pursue for diagnosis. Bilateral symmetry suggests a metabolic or endocrine problem, although I have seen food-allergic animals with symmetric hair-loss patterns. Alopecia with inflammation around the tail head, gluteal region, and perineum mandates an evaluation of the anal sac. Patchy hair loss, crusting of the ear margins, and patchy excoriations with intense pruritus are probably due to sarcoptic mange (Notoedres cati in the cat), but allergy, pemphigus, and other conditions can cause similar clinical signs. Even though few skin problems have pathognomonic signs or lesions, specific patterns are often associated with certain diseases and thus suggest, or at least exclude, specific diagnoses.

PHYSICAL EXAMINATION

Once the patient is on the examining table, run your fingers through the coat, feeling the quality and texture. See whether the patient is in good flesh or undernourished. Feel for crusts and scales, welts, and exudative patches. Weight loss or emaciation may be due to a metabolic problem or poor nutrition, but it may also be due to a loss of calories resulting from severe pruritus and the inability to rest properly.

EXAMINATION FORM

Owner _____

Patient Name _____ Species _____ Age _____ Sex _____

GENERAL APPEARANCE

Pruritus in office: Yes _____ No _____ Mild _____ Moderate _____ Severe _____

Comments _____

Describe hair coat _____

Hair loss: Yes _____ No _____ Describe pattern _____

Undercoat present: Yes _____ No _____ Coat dry _____ Scaly _____ Oily _____

SYSTEMATIC EXAMINATION

Eyes: Clear _____ If other, describe _____

Nose: Dry _____ Discharge _____ Describe _____

Lesions _____ Describe _____

Lesions on lips, muzzle, chin, face _____ Describe _____

Oral exam: Teeth _____ Mucosal lesions _____

Describe (with location) _____

Tonsils: Normal _____ Enlarged _____ Infected _____ Other _____

Ears: Normal _____ Discharge _____ Describe _____

Lesions _____ Describe _____

Lymph nodes: Normal _____ Enlarged _____ Location _____

Feet: Pustules _____ Inflammation _____ Foot pads cracked or crusting _____ Describe any

abnormalities _____

Lick granuloma(s) _____ Location _____

General condition of skin: Dry _____ Scaling _____ Crusts _____ Seborrhea _____ Pustules _

Papules _____ Nodules _____ Follicular plugs _____ Other _____

Location of lesions: Axillae _____ Inguinal area _____ Face _____

Other _____

Describe _____

Rectal:

Perianal region _____

Prostate: Normal _____ Abnormal _____ Describe _____

Anal sacs: Normal _____ Diseased _____ Describe sacs and content _____

Preputial discharge: Yes _____ No _____ Describe _____

Vaginal discharge: Yes _____ No _____ Describe _____

Heart: _____

Lungs: _____

Abdominal organ palpation: _____

LABORATORY PROCEDURES

Fecal_____ Scrapings _____ Urine _____ Heartworm _____ CBC/Diff. _____

Serum chem. _____ T_4 _____ T_3 _____ Cortisol _____ ANA _____

LE Prep _____ Serum electrophoresis _____ Immunoelectrophoresis _____ Coombs test _____

Abnormalities seen _____

Preliminary diagnosis _____

Final Diagnosis _____

Fig. 4–1. Examination form.

Skin

The skin of an allergic dog frequently feels moist or clammy and may be accompanied by seborrhea and hair loss, with a variable seborrheic odor. Because seborrhea, in itself, is a nonspecific finding, the most difficult part of the differential diagnosis is determining whether these findings are due to allergy or to other causes. Certain generalizations may be helpful in this regard:

1. Metabolic seborrheas are generally not particularly pruritic, unless the skin is dry or the pruritus is due to the secondary bacterial infection that usually accompanies seborrhea.
2. Nutritional seborrheas are usually dryer and more pruritic than allergic conditions.
3. Seborrheas due to allergy, immune-mediated disease, ectoparasites, and mange can be extremely pruritic.

If the patient has a full coat, clip off patches in different regions, to see what the underlying skin looks like. It is amazing how often an apparently healthy coat is hiding scales, crusts, welts, or a diffuse papular or nodular eruption.

Allergic Triad

Veterinary allergists often refer to the "allergic triad": face rubbing, axillary pruritus, and foot licking. These signs are apparently the analog of symptoms commonly seen in man. Children with rhinitis and itching nasal membranes, for example, often rub their hands across their noses in a gesture referred to as the "allergic salute." Allergic asthmatics frequently experience axillary pruritus accompanied by pruritus of the upper midback between the shoulder blades during an acute attack of asthma. Allergic patients will also occasionally develop pruritus of the palms and soles which can become intense, at times. Although clinical signs can occur anywhere on the body, these are the most common in dogs, and it is important not only to look for evidence of these signs when examining the patient, but also to question the client about them. Therefore, pay particular attention to the face and periorbital skin, check the feet, and examine the brisket and axillae because these are often affected in allergy and may be inflamed or excoriated.

When examining a patient, I like to start at the nose, progress down the back, auscult the chest, check the feet, and finish with a rectal examination. It really does not matter at which end one starts, as long as a regular procedure is followed.

Nose and Mouth

The planum of the nose is checked for cracking, irritation, loss of pigment, and ulceration, particularly at the mucocutaneous junction. Such lesions may be a result of allergic scratching or face rubbing, or they may signify something much more serious, such as an autoimmune disease. Look for nasal discharge and note whether it is serous or thick and whether nasal plugging is present. Flare-shaped hair loss over the dorsum of the nose, with its base at the border of the nasal planum, suggests hypothyroidism.

The mucosal surfaces of the patient's mouth are checked for erosive lesions that may also make one suspect an autoimmune disease. It is important not to overlook the tonsils because chronic tonsillitis can cause nasal discharge, coughing, or periodic vomiting, masquerading as allergy.

Eyes and Ears

Examine the eyes to see whether they are clear or whether conjunctivitis is visible. If discharge is present, note whether it is serous, mucoid, or purulent. A serous or mucoid discharge frequently accompanies allergic conjunctivitis or face rubbing. A serous discharge may also occur with infectious conjunctivitis, but infection usually produces a thicker discharge than allergy, and it is also frequently greenish or purulent.

Otitis is an often overlooked sign of allergy occurring much more frequently with food than with inhalant allergy. There is no definitive pattern; it can be unilateral or bilateral, a secondary infection may be present, and it may be the only sign of allergy in that patient. As a general rule, however, in allergic otitis the ear canals often have a doughy, inflamed moist appearance, and the pinnae may be doughy with a diffuse erythema that gradually fades toward the margins.

Auscultation

Although they are uncommon, allergic asthma, asthmatic bronchitis, and allergic tracheitis can occur. Therefore, it is important to auscult the patient and to listen for expiratory dyspnea or rales. The larynx and trachea should also be palpated and pinched lightly to see whether a stertorous cough is easily provoked. A honking cough, similar to that of infectious tracheobronchitis, can be due to allergy.

Parasite Evaluation

As one moves on to closer evaluation of the skin and hair coat, check for fleas, using a flea comb if necessary. Look for other ectoparasites, as well, and do multiple skin scrapings on both active and crusted lesions. Do not be fooled into thinking that because it looks like allergy or does not look like mange it does not have to be scraped.

I have a vivid memory of a dog that was presented to me with pruritus and a medical history highly suggestive of allergy. On close examination, I found one small patch of scaling seborrhea on the trunk. I had almost decided not to scrape the lesion, but did it anyway *out of force of habit*, not really expecting to find anything. To my surprise, I found a mass of cheyletiella mites swimming in my scraping oil. Although it is true that allergy was the dog's primary problem, how embarrassing it would have been to have her continue to scratch because I had missed a secondary parasite problem.

Remember that it is extremely rare, although not impossible, for two or more animals in the same household to suddenly develop an allergy and become pruritic within a short time of each other. If that occurs, look for parasites. If you do not find them, look again. Nothing can be more upsetting to a client than to have a pet treated for an allergy for months on end, only to find that the problem was really mange or some other parasitic infestation.

Feet

Look at the feet and check both the dorsal and volar interdigital webbing. These may be inflamed, exudative, or seborrheic. Interdig-ital cysts are also occasionally found because atopy often reduces resistance to infection. Be sure to scrape the toes and interdigital webbing; these are frequently the only places you may find demodectic mange, especially in older dogs. Podopyoderma and interdigital cysts are almost always secondary to some underlying problem and may indicate allergy, may represent an unrelated infection, or may be associated with demodex. Be sure to scrape, and scrape deeply, before eliminating demodex from consideration, especially in older dogs.

Abdomen

The lower abdomen, inguinal area, and medial thighs are frequent sites of allergic dermatitis, as are the flank folds and anterolateral aspects of the stifles. These commonly have a papulonodular eruption with alopecia.

While evaluating the abdomen, palpate deeply for tumors, enlargements, or other abnormalities. Feel the spleen and liver and check their borders for size and contour. Although such abnormalities are not often associated with skin or other allergic problems, they can indicate serious disease and should be corrected before beginning treatment for allergy. Check for intestinal gas and fluid levels and note whether flatulence is present. Lift the tail and look at the anus, to check for signs of diarrhea. Gastrointestinal changes are often associated with food allergy and are often overlooked, unless you are on the alert for it.

Rectum, Anal Sacs, and Lymph Nodes

Do a rectal examination evaluating the anal sacs and palpating the prostate in the male. If the prostate is enlarged or cystic, or if pus can be expressed, it must be treated. Not only can prostatic infections lead to debility, but also allergy can develop to foci of infection within the body.

The same is true for anal sacs. Anal sac infections can be a significant cause of dry, scaly skin, pruritus, and exudative dermatitis, especially over the posterior third of the body, although any part can be involved. Here, too, allergy to infected anal sac contents can develop, as discussed in more detail in Chapter 16.

Before completing the examination, remember to check the lymph nodes. The popliteal nodes are usually enlarged in patients with chronic skin irritation, probably as a result of superficial secondary infection. This is generally of no concern unless the other lymph nodes are enlarged, as well.

Finally, do not cut corners in the physical examination because the part you miss may be the key to the diagnosis.

LABORATORY EVALUATIONS

Criteria for laboratory data bases should be established, and, based on the patient's history and physical examination, test selections should be made. These can be divided into a *minimum database, a satisfactory database, and a complete database.* To this can be added special tests, as needed, such as thyroid, adrenal, and other endocrine studies, tests for immune-mediated diseases, allergy skin tests, and immunocompetency studies.

Minimum Database

A minimum database, although not recommended for most patients because of the limited information obtained, should contain, in addition to a thorough medical history, a fecal examination, skin scrapings, and a Wood's light examination.

Fecal Examination

Intestinal parasites, especially if the infestation is heavy, can cause loss of condition and a dry, thin coat. In addition, pruritus is occasionally seen in animals with intestinal parasitic infections.

Skin Scrapings

The value of skin scrapings should be self-evident. It is essential to know whether ectoparasites are present and whether they are the cause of the patient's problem.

Wood's Light Examination

Wood's light is only diagnostic for Microsporum canis. Although opinions vary among veterinarians, realistically it enables one to identify about 60% of the cases, depending on the skill of the individual veterinarian. Nevertheless, because fungal infections can vary in appearance and often do not look like fungal infections, this instrument should be used in every patient with a skin disorder presented for evaluation. The procedure is simple, the equipment is inexpensive, and if the result is positive, you have your diagnosis or at least a factor contributing to the diagnosis. Additional diagnostic evaluation is not usually required until the infection has been eliminated.

Satisfactory Database

To obtain a satisfactory database, one must add further tests to the minimum database. Integral to this is a complete blood count and differential, a serum chemistry panel, and a urinalysis. These tests not only give significant information, they also can help to identify important underlying medical problems, which may be more serious than the skin or allergy problem for which the patient is presented and thereby require prior attention.

Complete Blood Count and Differential

An eosinophilia, although not consistent, is sometimes seen in food allergy, especially in cats, and even, on occasion, in inhalant allergy. Eosinophils are often seen in nasal and conjunctival smears from people suffering with allergic rhinitis and conjunctivitis and help to confirm the diagnosis. Evidence supporting the value of such smears in animals is insufficient, but the procedure is quick and easy and would make a good research project for a clinician interested in the subject.

Microscopic Examination

If the Wood's light examination is negative, hair and skin samples should be examined microscopically for fungal elements, using either potassium hydroxide or fungal stains such as lactophenol cotton blue or pontamine sky blue. My personal preference is the stains because they are generally effective in staining and outlining fungal spores and hyphae in hair and on skin. Select the samples from the active, "leading edge" of the lesions, rather than from the healed center because the edge is the most likely location for finding actively growing dermatophytes.

Heartworm is an occasional cause of pruritus in some dogs. Therefore, unless the dog is receiving preventive medication and is tested regularly, a heartworm test should be done. Although metabolites from the adult may conceivably be responsible for the pruritus, the pruritic state is more likely a direct effect of the microfilaria on skin capillaries or nerve endings or of mediators released by immunocytes attacking the filaria.

Swab and impression smears can pack a lot of information onto a small slide and should always be made from weeping, draining, and ulcerative lesions. These office procedures do not take much time, can be prepared by a technician, and in many instances, establish or confirm your diagnosis. For example, Gram stains quickly tell you whether the lesion contains gram-positive or gram-negative bacteria, thereby suggesting which classes of antibacterials will be most effective for treatment while you wait for a culture and sensitivity report. Quick stains, such as Difquick, are simple to use and can be helpful in arriving at a diagnosis/treatment plan. When eosinophils are found in blood smears or in nasal or ocular discharges, allergy is the most likely cause. Impression smears can help to identify deep fungi and pathogenic yeasts, as well as tumor cells, thereby adding invaluable information to the differential diagnosis.

Complete Database

To arrive at a complete database, add cultures, biopsies, allergy skin tests, and other special tests where indicated.

Cultures

Whether culturing for bacteria or fungal infections, it is important to subculture mixed colony growth and to identify each organism individually. When culturing bacteria, run antibiotic sensitivity tests on each subcultured species. Unless you are an experienced bacteriologist and mycologist, the cultures should be done in a commercial laboratory, with instructions to make and identify individual isolates.

From a practical point of view, it is best to use a veterinary laboratory for bacterial cultures and sensitivities because human laboratories use many antibiotics in their sensitivity spectrum that are available only for human use or are best suited for use in hospitalized patients. This situation can be a particular problem when culturing ears because human laboratories generally do not test for topical antibiotics, and the report will list sensitivity tests for antibiotics unavailable in a clinically useful form.

One other caution: Many organisms can be dangerous and should be handled only under a laboratory hood or under conditions safe for you and your staff. This is another reason to leave cultures in the hands of professionals.

Biopsy

Performing biopsies on every skin case would be academically desirable, but economically and clinically impractical. Biopsies, which provide a picture of the skin at the microscopic level, often only suggest probable diagnoses. Therefore, it is reasonable to withhold biopsies for most skin problems initially and to perform them if the response to treatment is unsatisfactory. A biopsy would then either confirm your original diagnosis or point you in another direction. Biopsies are indicated on the first evaluation, however, in lesions that you suspect are due to either autoimmune or malignant disease. They would also be indicated in any condition that has a strange or unusual appearance or has not been seen before.

One additional area in which biopsies can be invaluable is in the diagnosis of demodicosis, particularly in the Shar-Pei. Perhaps because of the mucinous character of the skin of this breed, mites are often found in skin biopsies, but not on multiple, deep skin scrapings. This happens occasionally in other dogs, as well. I have seen uncommon cases of demodicosis that failed to respond to treatment, yet gradually became negative based on skin scrapings. Skin biopsies from these same dogs occasionally showed demodex deep in the follicles. Although no rational explanation exists for the inability to express the mites, even by pinching and deep scraping, it does demonstrate that because something is not readily seen, does not mean it is not there. Every diagnostic tool available should be used in evaluating and treating a patient.

Allergy Skin Tests

Allergy skin testing is discussed in detail in Chapter 10. In summary, however, tests should be used only when the patient's history, physical examination, and other diagnostic procedures have convinced you that the condition is, in fact, an *inhalant* allergy. This testing is not recommended for the diagnosis of food or contact allergies.

Special Tests

Thyroid and adrenal function tests are probably the most frequently performed special tests. Unfortunately, they are often run unnecessarily, particularly thyroid function tests, creating an unnecessary expense for the patient's owner. These tests are not intended for use as a "fishing trip" when the veterinarian does not know what to do next. In-stead, they should be run only when all clinical indicators suggest that either or both organs are not functioning properly. Thyroid function tests, in particular, can be affected by many factors, including medications taken by the patient, hyperadrenocorticism, febrile illness, anorexia, and cachexia.

For a detailed discussion of the clinical signs and interpretation of laboratory procedures for use in thyroid and adrenal conditions, the reader is referred to any complete text on endocrinology and general dermatology.

A lupus erythematosus (LE) preparation and antinuclear antibody (ANA) tests are indicated for the diagnosis of lupus erythematosus. Neither of these tests is absolutely diagnostic, however, and both false-positive and false-negative results may occur. Therefore, a final diagnosis can only be made when all the information has been assembled, including the patient's history, clinical findings, laboratory data, and biopsies for both routine histopathology and fluorescent antibody.

Clinical Signs

There is a perception among most veterinary clinicians, including some veterinary dermatologists, that allergy involves only the skin. Although it is true that the skin is the principal target organ in both canine and feline allergy, it is far from the only organ system. Allergy can also involve the upper and lower respiratory tract, ocular tissue, the gastrointestinal tract, the nervous system, and the genitourinary tract. Ectodermally derived tissues, such as skin and mucous membranes, are probably the principal sites of allergic reactions, although other tissues may be involved as well.

SKIN

Allergy-associated *skin* lesions can be found anywhere on the body, although the predilection seems to be for periorbital skin, the axillae and antecubital areas, the popliteal region, the foot pads, and the lower abdomen. In white-faced dogs, such as the Dalmatian and English bulldog, fiery erythema around the muzzle and eyelids is considered almost pathognomonic for allergy (Fig. 5–1).

Among the early skin lesions is a pruritic papulonodular eruption that can be localized, patchy, or generalized (Fig. 5–2). As the condition progresses, a patchy or diffuse erythema becomes more prominent and pruritus intensifies, resulting in lichenification, self-induced abrasions, excoriations, and ulcerations (Fig. 5–3). Progressive changes ranging from fine dander and scales to seborrheic plaques and crusts often occur in allergic dermatitis. This sequence, in turn, is followed by hair loss, which can be extensive. The lichenified skin thickens and becomes pigmented, and the seborrhea becomes progressively more severe and foul smelling. Alopecia, pruritus, and hyperkeratosis are often so severe that the condition is virtually impossible to distinguish from sarcoptic mange. Because any change from normal promotes

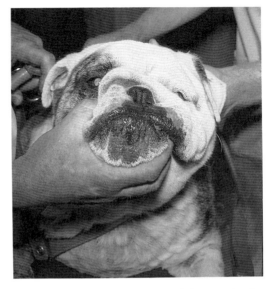

Fig. 5–1. Allergic erythema around the muzzle of an English bulldog.

increased bacterial colonization of the skin, seborrheic lesions are almost always accompanied by secondary infections, which can cause additional pruritus and inflammation, thus aggravating an already aggravated skin.

Exudative dermatitis, the so-called "hot spots" (Fig. 5–4), is a common condition that essentially represents the end stage of a localized pruritic wheal that has been self-trau-

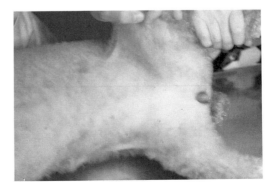

Fig. 5–2. Allergic papulonodular eruption in a poodle.

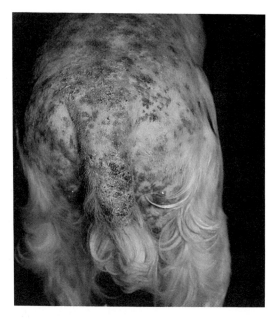

Fig. 5–3. Allergic seborrhea in an English setter.

matized through licking, biting, and scratching. Such lesions are usually found on medium- or long-haired dogs, although short-haired dogs are occasionally affected, as well. As the lesion is traumatized and spread, there is serous exudation, accompanied by matting of the overlying hair, explaining the predilection of exudative dermatitis for longer-haired dogs. This condition is followed by superficial bacterial infection, which causes more pruritus, thus perpetuating the cycle. Effective treatment is usually possible by simply clipping and

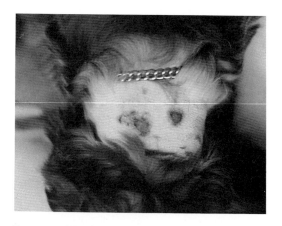

Fig. 5–4. Allergic exudative dermatitis in a golden retriever.

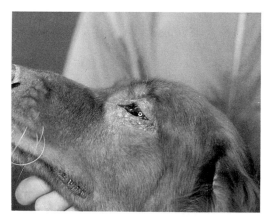

Fig. 5–5. Allergic periorbital alopecia in a golden retriever.

cleaning the affected area, washing it with a mild soap, patting it dry, and allowing it to be exposed to the air.

The progression of lesions just described really represents a "worst-case scenario." Because clinical cases rarely follow textbook courses, one may see any combination of clinical signs, ranging from mild to severe. The severity of the case has little relationship to the response to treatment: some severe cases respond well, whereas other, milder cases may respond poorly.

EYES

Ocular lesions consist essentially of conjunctivitis and blepharitis that is sometimes severe enough to cause blepharospasm and light sensitivity. A serous or mucoid ocular discharge is common and may cause inflammation of the skin over the medial canthus with periorbital alopecia, inflammation, and crusting (Fig. 5–5).

Allergic conjunctivitis can be pruritic, causing the cat or dog to rub or scratch the face and eyes, with resulting periorbital inflammation, hair loss, and excoriations. The patient is often presented with a band of alopecia around the eyes, sometimes extending over the face and nose, that must be distinguished from pemphigus, discoid lupus, and other immune-mediated diseases.

EARS

Although allergic otitis and pinnal edema are commonly associated with food allergy,

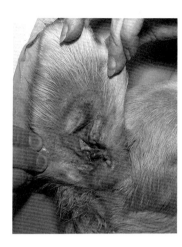

Fig. 5–6.   Allergic otitis in a golden retriever.

they are often seen with inhalant allergy, as well (Fig. 5–6). In people, itching of the tympanum and nasopharynx can cause significant discomfort, and I strongly suspect that it can also be a severe problem in dogs. It would be difficult to prove, of course, but when one observes how some allergic dogs tear at their throats and the bases of their ears, it is as though they were trying to reach back into the throat, or down the ear canal, in an attempt to relieve the itch.

RESPIRATORY SYSTEM

Upper Respiratory Tract

Even though some veterinary allergists do not include *upper respiratory changes* among their clinical signs of allergy, in my experience these changes often occur. These include allergic tracheitis, sinus snorting, sneezing, and nasal discharge.

Allergic Tracheitis

Clinically, it is virtually impossible to distinguish allergic tracheitis from infectious tracheobronchitis. Both are easily provoked, both are characteristically harsh and honking, and both can be prolonged. The differential diagnosis is based on the patient's medical history and the therapeutic trial. Although both the allergic and infectious forms have a sudden onset, dogs with allergic tracheitis usually have no history of boarding, grooming, or exposure to other potentially infected dogs. Treatment consists of admin-

istering a short-acting parenteral corticosteroid and an injectable antihistamine. The patient usually responds in about 6 hours, and the improvement may last for several days. If allergen exposure continues and the cough recurs, an oral antihistamine at full therapeutic dose usually keeps the condition under control.

Sinus Snorting

Sinus snorting, often referred to as a "reverse sneeze," is another clinical sign often caused by allergy, although there can be other causes as well. Clinically, attacks may occur once in several months or many times a day. Typically, the dog stands with head down and forelegs slightly spread, while making strong inspiratory motions in an apparent attempt to draw mucus plugs from the turbinates into the nasopharynx, where they can then be swallowed.

The exact cause is uncertain, but the nature of the syndrome suggests that thick mucus forming in the sinuses drains into the nasal turbinates where it lodges as plugs, either irritating the dog or causing mild respiratory distress. The frequency of attacks often parallels that of sinus attacks in man. Although zoographic studies have not been done, I suspect that the incidence is higher in areas where sinus disease is also high in man.

Attacks usually respond well to decongestant nasal drops administered 2 to 3 times daily. When attacks are frequent or severe, oral antihistamines may be effective. If not, preparations containing 0.5 mg prednisolone, 25 mg diphenhydramine (or other suitble antihistamine), and 15 to 30 mg ephedrine sulfate, 2 to 3 times daily, have been beneficial. This preparation is not commercially available and must be compounded by the veterinarian or a local pharmacy.

Nasal Discharges and Sneezing

Nasal discharge and sneezing, although not major clinical signs, occur more often than generally recognized. Unfortunately, this information is frequently overlooked in patients presented for the treatment of dermatitis or other allergic problems, and the patient's owner usually does not offer the information unless questioned. These signs respond reasonably well to antihistamines and nose drops.

Nonetheless, it is not enough merely to assume that sneezing and discharge are "probably allergic," without a careful examination. The nasal passages are difficult to visualize grossly or even radiographically and may require fiberoptic examination for a final diagnosis. Sneezing and discharge can be caused by tumors, foreign objects, or infections. Therefore, cytologic examination for abnormal cells and bacteria should be performed and nasal discharges cultured, if indicated. If the patient does not respond to treatment within a reasonable period and if it is not possible to perform a more extensive examination, the patient should be referred to a university or specialty practice for a diagnostic and therapeutic consultation.

Lower Respiratory Tract

Allergic manifestations in the *lower respiratory tract* are not common, but asthma and asthmatic bronchitis do occasionally occur. The first proved case of inhalant allergy in a dog was diagnosed in 1939 by a physician allergist in Milwaukee, who observed that his dog developed severe asthma every August, concurrent with the onset of the ragweed season. Skin tests for ragweed pollen were positive, and a subsequent course of immunotherapy provided excellent allergy control for the remainder of the dog's life.

I have seen occasional cases of asthma and allergic bronchitis, but the dog I remember the best is one I saw shortly after I became interested in allergy. Every year, she would start to cough on or about August 15 and would become progressively worse through mid-September, when the asthma would improve gradually before finally disappearing after the first hard frost. She, too, gave a 4 + reaction to ragweed and had an excellent response to immunotherapy with ragweed antigen.

Asthma as a primary clinical manifestation of allergy is unusual; most dogs with asthma, allergic bronchitis, or other lower respiratory problems usually have other, more common allergic signs for which they are presented for treatment, so the respiratory problem is often overlooked. This situation highlights a problem that continues to plague veterinary allergy. As long as veterinarians and clients alike continue to view allergy as an exclusively dermatologic disorder, other clinical signs will continue to be overlooked or misdiagnosed.

Cats appear to develop asthma more often than dogs, with foods and cat litter dust the most common offenders. Attacks tend to be short-lived, clearing spontaneously without treatment. If attacks are prolonged, or if they cause undue distress in either the dog or cat, one or two short sprays of albuterol or isoproterenol in a metered-dose nebulizer, during inspiration, will usually bring quick relief.

One final word about asthma. Even though it may not be a common clinical sign, asthma can be induced in most dogs with inhalant allergy if they are placed in an aerosol chamber into which high concentrations of allergens are insufflated.

GASTROINTESTINAL TRACT

Gastrointestinal signs are usually associated with food allergy, but they can also occur with inhalant allergy. Clinical signs can begin within minutes of eating the offending food, or they may not occur for 24 hours or longer. Such signs vary widely and include eructation, flatulence, vomiting, and diarrhea, which can be profuse and bloody. Gastrointestinal signs are often cyclic, even when the diet is unvaried. A seeming tolerance may exist for up to several weeks before the sudden onset of clinical signs. Several hours to days of distress, often unresponsive to treatment, are followed by a return to normal. Why this should happen is not clear. It has been postulated, however, that in the case of a low-grade food sensitivity, a state of "progressive antigen loading" may exist in which occasional small feedings would cause no problems, whereas frequent feedings allow enough antigen buildup to elicit an allergic reaction. Although this theory leaves many questions unanswered, it will have to suffice until a better one is developed.

A syndrome one sees occasionally, allergic hemorrhagic enteritis, is characterized by the sudden onset of a profusely bloody diarrhea that smells like an open sewer. The dog, however, does not seem to be in any particular distress, is playful, and enters the examining room alert and wagging its tail. The dog has no history of ingesting foreign objects or possible poisons, and on examination shows no evidence of obstruction or foreign body. Following rectal examination, one often finds strings or clumps of mucus with streaks of blood on the gloved finger. These patients usually respond dramatically, within 6 hours, to a single dose of a short-acting parenteral steroid and an injectable antihistamine, such as diphenhydramine.

Before starting treatment, one should be confident in the diagnosis. A complete history and thorough physical examination are essential, and radiographs should be taken if there is any indication of intestinal obstruction. Unless the precipitating agent is obvious, the owner should be instructed to review carefully everything the dog ingested during the prior 48 hours and to record everything that was new, different, or prepared in a different manner. If the patient has recurrent bouts, the owner should keep a complete and accurate diet diary and should attempt to find a common factor.

Genitourinary and neurologic disorders are also generally overlooked as possible allergic disorders by most veterinary allergists and dermatologists. Yet many case reports in the human literature implicate food and other allergens as etiologic agents in a variety of these disorders, such as enuresis, behavior problems, and infertility. Admittedly, this subject is controversial, but it should at least make one explore an allergic basis for a recurrent or unresponsive condition of which the definitive cause is uncertain. My own experience, as well as that of others, bears out this approach.

GENITOURINARY TRACT

Genitourinary signs, which either go unrecognized or are much less common than those associated with other organ systems, are usually caused by foods or other noninhalant allergens.

Although immunologic studies have not been conducted to confirm an allergic basis, allergy-associated cystitis has been seen in both man and, occasionally, dogs. The diagnosis is based on the patient's history and response to therapeutic trials. To date, all cases seen in my practice and reported to me by others have been associated with food and can be relieved or provoked by dietary manipulation. Admittedly, this does not prove that cystitis is a result of allergy or is even associated with an immunologic reaction, but the presumptive criteria for allergy are strong.

Specific immune reactions involving the reproductive tract have been described in men and may result in infertility because of antisperm antibodies, sperm-immobilizing antibodies, or a sperm antigen cell-mediated immune response. Asthma, urticaria, and angioedema, all commonly associated with Type I sensitivity reactions, have also been reported in women following sexual intercourse. Skin test reactions to their partner's seminal proteins were positive, and some improvement occurred following immunotherapy.

In animals, antisperm antibody has also been found in cattle and may cause infertility in this species. Orchitis resulting from injury, in any species, or Brucella canis in male dogs, may induce autoantibodies to their own sperm that cause infertility. A Type I or Type IV autoallergy to testosterone, estrogen, or progesterone is occasionally seen in dogs and is accompanied by pruritus, which is often intense, a papulonodular eruption, and erythema.

The ability to develop antibodies against sperm and reproductive hormones can be important in population control, and it is the basis for much current research in animal contraception.

CENTRAL NERVOUS SYSTEM

Neurologic signs are variable and, again, occur mostly in food allergy. I have seen patients with food allergy-associated convulsive seizures, and so have other clinicians. At the annual meeting of the American Veterinary Medical Association in Washington, D.C., in 1982, Dr. Jay Collins of Houston, Texas, reported on three cases of epileptiform convulsions caused by food.[1] All three animals in this report responded to a change in diet, and in all three, convulsions returned during dietary challenges. Many, much more subtle neurologic changes are also associated with food allergy. When food-allergic animals are fasted or are otherwise relieved of the offending food, the most common comments made by their owners are: "he seems so much more relaxed," "she sleeps so much better at night," "her temperament has improved—she's not as snappy," "he's more tolerant." Admittedly, these effects may be indirect, but they are associated with the allergy nonetheless.

Finally, although all veterinary internists and immunologists recognize the many immune-mediated diseases that can affect virtually every organ, little investigative effort has gone into the possibility of allergic reactions affecting these same organs. Except for the dermatologic reactions and, to a lesser extent, gastrointestinal changes, allergic reactions have not been studied extensively in animals. Part of the problem is that veterinary allergy is still "the new kid on the block," having gained acceptance and respectability only in recent years. When I first became interested in allergic diseases in the early 1950s, no self-respecting academician would admit that it was anything more than an aberration, a medical curiosity. Unfortunately, even though allergy has now gained full recognition as a major clinical problem, most veterinarians, including most veterinary dermatologists, still consider allergy a dermatologic disease. As noted at the beginning of this chapter, until this attitude changes, little foward movement can occur in the identification and study of allergic reactions involving other organ systems.

REFERENCE

1. Collins, J.R.: Food hypersensitivity-induced canine seizures. Presented at the 119th Annual Meeting of the American Veterinary Medical Association, Washington, D.C., July 20, 1982.

6 ‖ *Predisposing Factors in Allergy*

The essence of allergy may be the allergen/antibody/mast cell reaction, but many factors play a role in the development or aggravation of the allergic response. Primary among these is heredity.

GENETIC FACTORS

Although it certainly is possible for genes to mutate so an individual with no allergic forebears may suddenly become sensitive, an allergic individual typically has at least one allergic parent. One does not inherit an allergy to a specific agent from one's ancestors; rather, one inherits the ability to develop an allergy *to something.* For example, an individual may have one parent with a sensitivity to ragweed and one with an allergy to maple pollen. Yet the offspring, who is now genetically programmed for allergy, may react to the same antigen(s) as the parents or to a totally different group.

ENVIRONMENTAL FACTORS

Many environmental factors influence the onset or severity of an allergic reaction. Although not specifically allergenic in themselves, these factors can influence the antigen load or physiologic priming of the allergic patient.

Heating Systems

A good example is a household hot-air heating system. In addition to the extra antigen load such systems place in the environment, as discussed further in Chapter 8, they also dry the skin and mucous membranes. Dry skin increases pruritus in an already pruritic animal, whereas low humidification of mucosal surfaces increases reactivity and irritability, making it easier for antigens to pass through these surfaces.

Humidifiers

Proper humidification, therefore, is extremely important with central hot-air heat or with individual room space heaters. Humidifiers are not a panacea, however, and they, too, can present problems. Although inadequate humidification is undesirable, too much moisture leads to mold growth on interior surfaces, again increasing the antigenic potential. If humidifiers are not emptied and cleaned or, in the case of in-line furnace humidifiers, not maintained properly, mold will grow within the system and will be distributed continually during operating cycles.

Air-Filtration Systems

Good air-filtration systems are also important because unfiltered or improperly filtered air increases allergen concentration and exposure. Among the filters, fiberglass mesh is probably the poorest; it allows the largest range of particle sizes to pass through and thereby increases the potential for exposure in sensitive individuals.

Until the last several years, the electrostatic precipitator was considered the best filter for ordinary household use, especially when accompanied by an in-line pre- and afterfilter. Electrostatic precipitators are available as either individual room units or as furnace units installed in the return airflow duct. These filters contain charged plates that attract and precipitate oppositely charged particles as the air flow is forced through the filter.

The latest advance in filter design is the HEPA type, an acronym for high-efficiency particulate air filters, which can even trap particles under one micron in diameter. Because of the amount of force required to propel air through the dense filter, these filters were not suitable for in-furnace use until recently and were only available as room units. A furnace unit has now been designed to be used with central hot-air and air-conditioning units. A combination of HEPA and electrostatic precipitators would probably be an ideal combination for in-line furnace air filtration.

The most important thing to remember about any air-filtration system is that it must be kept clean to be efficient. If a disposable filter is used, it must be changed at frequent intervals and before it becomes so clogged that it is virtually useless. If washable filters are used, they should be inspected and cleaned regularly, to maintain maximum efficiency.

Indoor Plants and Shrubbery Beds

Nothing is lovelier than a house full of lush, green plants or a finely manicured lawn with deep, well-mulched shrubbery beds. To the mold-sensitive individual, however, such beauty can spell disaster.

Potting soil and shrubbery beds provide an ideal environment for mold growth because they supply both moisture and organic matter on which to thrive. The beds can be particularly disastrous because they provide not only an environment for growth, but also a place for dogs and cats to dig, stirring up massive clouds of microscopic, allergenic mold spores. Mulch and leaf piles, decaying grass clippings, or any accumulation of organic matter can provide a sufficiently high concentration of mold spores to provoke an allergic attack in an otherwise quiescent, but mold-sensitive, patient.

Weather

Weather can trigger the onset or increase the severity of an allergic problem in many ways. Cool, moist, and damp weather provides ideal growing conditions for many molds and triggers the release of untold millions of spores into the air. Warm, bright, airy days, on the other hand, are ideal conditions for the release and distribution of many plant pollens. Cooling air at night promotes the settling of allergenic particles, thereby increasing the concentration near the floor where pets lie. As air warms, on the other hand, it rises, producing convection currents that cause allergens to rise and circulate in the air.

Low barometric pressures force allergenic particles, as well as industrial and other air pollutants, closer to the ground and increase the potential allergenic load. High barometric pressures are more likely to keep the particles floating higher and longer, distributing them over a much wider area.

Strong winds drive particles toward the allergic individual with greater intensity and so increase the likelihood of allergen contact and an allergic reaction. The Santa Ana winds of southern California are a good example of this phenomenon. Every allergic individual in the area knows the winds are blowing long before they appear in the weather reports.

Parasites

Fleas, ticks, lice, rhabditis (Pelodera strongyloides) and hookworm larvae (creeping eruption) can initiate an allergic response to the individual parasite, but no substantive evidence suggests that these parasites act as the initiating stimulus for an inhalant, food, or other allergic reaction. Some veterinarians have speculated that flea-bite dermatitis, in particular, may be a predisposing factor in inhalant allergic disease. As with other parasites, there is no strong evidence for this, although it is possible, of course, that flea allergen may alter immunoglobulin E (IgE) suppressor T cells while stimulating IgE production. The altered T-supressor cells could then lead to uninhibited IgE production and the induction of allergy. For now, however, this can only be considered speculative.

It is easy to understand the rationale behind this assumption. In many areas of the country, where fleas are generally not a problem throughout the year, the beginning of the flea season and the inhalant allergy season coincide. Therefore, as the dog starts scratching, fleas are the first thing seen, and the condition becomes, by extension, a flea-bite problem. When the pet is later found to have allergies, most owners, and frequently the veterinarian, assume that "it all started with the fleas." At best, flea-bite inflammation may prime the skin, enhancing the irritative inhalant allergic reaction, but one has to question seriously whether fleas can be responsible for converting the nonallergic individual to an allergic state.

Geographic Factors

Living in a northern, temperate, or semi-tropical latitude, in the desert, plains, or mountains, in marshy, swampy regions, or along a rain belt can make a difference in the type of pollens, molds, or environmental agents one looks for when determining the cause of allergy.

Fleas, for example, as discussed in Chapter 15, enjoy low altitudes and a hot, humid climate. Therefore, flea-bite allergy would be uncommon in the desert or at altitudes above 5000 feet.

The desert itself was once considered a safe haven for aeroallergen sufferers. Although some allergens are certainly indigenous to the area, they are limited to occasional mold spores and a few pollinating plants. Sparse vegetation and open spaces dilute the already low allergen load even further. With urbanization and increased population of desert communities, however, people brought their home-town environment with them and tried to create a landscape typical of the one they left, thereby introducing or increasing the very allergens they were trying to escape. It is unfortunate that many parts of the desert are no longer safe havens for allergy sufferers, and the medical practice of allergy treatment for both animals and man has blossomed.

Temperate and semitropical environments have longer allergy seasons than colder regions. As one travels farther south and along the Gulf coast and into Texas and California, seasons are gradually lost. Eventually, one finds just one continuous allergy season, as one pollinating plant follows another and molds sporulate continuously.

Low-lying river delta regions, marshy, swampy regions, and rain belts, typical of those found in the Pacific Northwest, are high mold-spore areas. The high atmospheric moisture, coupled with a temperate to warm climate, provides excellent growing conditions for molds. Therefore, molds are much more important allergens under these geographic and climatic conditions than in dryer regions.

Anticipated antigen load differs, based on whether one lives in mountainous regions or on the open plains. The higher the elevation, the sparser the vegetation and the lower the allergen load. Reduced thermal updrafts and the barrier protection of mountain slopes are also protective. In the plains states, however, without the protective windbreaks provided by mountains, spores and pollens have been estimated to blow for up to 500 miles, making it virtually impossible to escape them.

Because the plains states are the grain belt of the nation, in addition to the usual pollen and molds associated with indigenous trees and weeds are other allergens found in higher concentration than elsewhere. The most important of these are rusts, smuts, and granary dust, which should always be included in any test program in the midwest or in any other section in which they occur in high concentration.

Although much of the preceding is covered in more detail in Chapters 7 and 8, I have tried to stress here that many subtle factors affect the development of allergy and the onset of an allergic attack.

Aeroallergens

Technically, any particulate matter carried in the air that ultimately is inhaled and is capable of causing an allergic reaction could be classified as an aeroallergen. When the allergist speaks of aeroallergens, however, he usually refers to weed, grass, or tree pollens and airborne mold spores. Other particulate matter, such as dust, feathers, insect particles, wool, and kapok, are relegated to the environmental group, and these are dealt with in Chapter 8. To confuse matters even more, although both aeroallergens and environmental agents are inhaled, one commonly sees only the environmental agents referred to as inhalants in the literature.

Clinically, the only difference between inhalant and environmental allergy is that inhalant allergies are usually seasonal, whereas environmental allergies are nonseasonal. These distinctions become fuzzy, however, in warm climates where mold spores and varying pollens are almost always in the air. Even some environmental allergens, such as dust, vary in concentration, being higher during cold weather when the heating system is turned on than during the summer months.

Moreover, terminology is often far from precise. For example, ragweed pollinosis is the most common cause of hay fever in man in North America. The term is an unfortunate misnomer because the condition is not caused by hay and fever rarely occurs. It has become so firmly entrenched in the medical lexicon, however, that it is not likely to be replaced soon.

Because inhalant allergy is a recently accepted phenomenon in animals, and hay fever signs are an uncommon feature of the disease, we must hope that veterinarians will not adopt terminology that is not truly descriptive of the clinical syndrome. The acronym AID, although unofficial, has become the generally accepted designation for inhalant allergy in animals. Unfortunately, as

originally defined, it referred specifically to allergic inhalant dermatitis. Because respiratory and other clinical signs can be associated with inhalant allergy, I would urge the Academy of Veterinary Allergy to redefine AID as allergic inhalant *disease,* to be more descriptive of all the clinical signs possible in inhalant allergy.

Although one may treat allergy without knowing much about the natural history of allergens, a much higher level of understanding of the disease can be achieved by knowing something about the relative allergenicity, geographic distribution, and cross-reactivity of plants and molds.

POLLEN

Antigenic Components

Pollen grains and mold spores can be complex structures, containing multiple protein molecules with antigenic potentials ranging from nonimmunogenic to highly allergenic. The importance of isolating the most antigenic fractions is obvious; the more specific the allergen, the more accurate the diagnosis and the more effective the treatment. Because research in this field is new, the significant allergens have not been determined for most species. A notable exception is ragweed, from which a highly antigenic fraction, designated antigen E, has been isolated. This antigen is generally believed to be the most significant, but not the only, antigen in ragweed allergenic for man. At this time, we do not know whether the fractions identified in ragweed and other pollen as the significant allergens for man are the same ones responsible for allergic reactions in the dog and cat. Considering the similarity in the pathobiology of allergy in dog and man, however, it is probable that the significant fractions will be of equal importance in both species.

The ultimate goals, then, in the immunotherapy of allergy would be to determine which of the multiple protein molecules are the actual sensitizers, to isolate those fractions, and to treat patients specifically. Until it becomes possible to test and treat only with highly specific antigens, we must be content to use extracts known to be mixtures of proteins that may vary from batch to batch in both proportional ratios and concentrations. Despite their shortcomings, currently available antigens are still capable of eliciting excellent testing and treatment responses.

Cross-Reactivity

Although cross-reactivity may be found in pollen of closely related species, this is variable and inconstant. Grass species, for example, are probably among the most cross-reactive of all plants. Trees, on the other hand, have little cross-reactivity, except in closely related species. As discussed later, this variability can be important when deciding whether to use mixtures of allergens for skin testing.

Atmospheric Dispersion

The natural history of wind-pollinated, or anemophilous, plants makes fascinating reading, but an exhaustive account is beyond the scope of this book. Most people think of flowers only as brightly colored, decorative, aromatic structures, designed to attract insects, and do not realize that "nonflowering" plants have flowers, as well. Simply put, flowers are reproductive organs, containing pollen, seed-producing organs, or both. Unlike insect-pollinated, or entomophilous, flowers, those of plants producing airborne pollen are rarely colorful and are usually small and unisexual, with the male, or pollen-producing, flowers separated from the female seed producers.

To be clinically significant, pollen must be light and wind-borne, it must contain potent allergenic fractions, and it must reach high atmospheric concentrations. Because pollen from brightly flowering plants is usually heavy and sticky and is carried by insects, it rarely causes allergy. The amounts that do become airborne are usually of no consequence. When flowering plants grow in profusion, however, enough pollen may become dispersed locally into the air to cause a prob-

lem. These plants may also present a potential problem for dogs and cats, who stick their noses directly into the flowers or who sniff the ground where pollen has fallen and take long drafts of the potentially allergenic particles. Dogs and cats probably have a greater potential for developing allergies to flowering plants than man because of this sniffing, "vacuuming" process.

Not all wind-pollinated plants have the same potential for allergenicity, and some are apparently not allergenic at all. Pine pollen, for example, can reach high concentrations in the atmosphere, yet apparently causes little allergy in man. Whether the same is true for dogs is uncertain at this time.

As discussed in Chapter 6, weather can greatly influence the distribution and concentration of aeroallergens. Rain washes the atmosphere clean of pollen, while promoting release and rapidly increasing concentrations of some mold spores. Light, airy days, on the other hand, increase release and concentration of many types of pollen. The reason is probably that pollen, before release, is moist and heavy. Within minutes of exposure to sunshine, however, the pollen dehydrates and loses up to 50% of its weight, enhancing its ability to be carried on the wind. Different plants release their pollen at different times of the day. This is probably partially dependent on climatic factors.

The time of biologic release of pollen has not been studied for all allergenic species, but release of ragweed pollen, for example, is highest in the early morning.

Weather has other influences on aeroallergens. Warm days, with plenty of rain during the growing season, stimulate the growth and density of vegetation and increase the potential pollen load. Moreover, the stronger the wind, the higher the increase in atmospheric pollen concentration and the greater the distance it travels.

Pollen and Mold Counts

Important aids in determining which aeroallergens are present in high enough concentrations in the atmosphere to cause problems are the weekly air-sample reports available from companies producing allergenic extracts and the major regional hospitals around the country. Because the time of pollination varies among different geographic and climatic regions, one must use pollen and mold counts from local sources. Even then, conditions within a specific locale or neighborhood can differ from the regional count, depending on the vegetation in the immediate area. Because individual counts from each patient's environment are impractical, if not impossible, regional counts help to provide a general picture of the most probable aeroallergens in the area.

Pollen and mold sampling techniques vary, and detailed discussion is unnecessary here. For the interested reader, information on approved techniques and instrumentation is available from the American Academy of Allergy and Clinical Immunology and from texts on human allergy.

Clinical Significance

Much of what I say about aeroallergens is extrapolated from information in man or is based on personal experience. It must be emphasized that the critical studies necessary to positively identify specific molds and pollen as animal sensitizers have not been done, although the clinical and presumptive evidence is more than satisfactory. Moreover, a positive skin-test reaction is not proof that a particular antigen is responsible for a clinical problem. It only indicates the presence of skin-sensitizing antibody, which may or may not have clinical significance, and findings must be correlated with the patient's history, when possible.

Unfortunately, one cannot prove sensitivity without housing the pet in an environmentally controlled chamber or periodically challenging it in an aerosol chamber. Such a chamber would be insufflated with individual molds and pollens, while one observed the patient for reactions. Because this process would be extremely costly and time consuming, as well as impractical, certain assumptions must be made.

1. Because the pathophysiology of allergy in the dog is so similar to that in man, except for the target organ, allergenic agents are probably the same, or similar, in both species.

2. Because virtually no environment has only one species of aeroallergen present in the atmosphere at any one time, the patient's medical history is of little value in identifying individual molds or pollen species. The patient's history is extremely important, however, in identifying the allergen season(s) during which the patient has a problem.

3. Because positive reactions to several different trees, weeds, or molds may be found, and because one cannot determine which of the reactions, if any, is clinically significant, it is necessary to treat the patient for all positive reactions.

4. As little as can be said for the dog in this regard, even less can be said for the cat. Other than a few limited skin-testing and treatment studies, little is known about inhalant allergy in this species. To my knowledge, immunoglobulin E (IgE) has still not been isolated, although we presume that it exists. Because skin testing and immunotherapy apparently work in the limited number of cats in which they have been tried, I see no reason not to continue testing and treating these animals while awaiting more definitive information.

TREES

Pollination Times

Trees are the first plants to pollinate in the continental United States, except in parts of Florida and Texas, where some grasses pollinate throughout the year. In most states, pollination begins by mid-March and rarely extends beyond May. The length of the total pollination season depends on the latitude at which trees grow, the time at which the weather usually starts to turn warm, and the number of anemophilous tree species growing in a specific geographic area. The time when individual trees begin to pollinate is genetically determined and depends on when they arise from dormancy, relative to reaching the proper ambient temperature, and their normal flowering period.

Thus, trees may begin pollinating in Texas in mid-December, in Louisiana by the first of January, and in Georgia and Alabama by mid-January. Florida, on the other hand, has a short tree-pollination period, in spite of its subtropical climate, probably because of the small number of wind-pollinated tree species in most of the state.

Pine Sensitivity

Pine appears to be an exception to all the rules about allergenically important species. Although pine pollen fulfills the criteria for potential allergenicity, being both abundant and lightweight for rapid atmospheric distribution, it is not considered to be clinically significant in man. Whether the same is also true for the dog is uncertain, although some veterinarians who test patients with pine pollen not only obtain positive skin-test results, but also believe their patients respond well to immunotherapy.

Therefore, in spite of the lack of evidence for pine sensitivity, if you live in an area with a high pine density and have patients that either worsen when pine pollen counts are high or do not respond as well to immunotherapy as expected, empiric testing for pine pollen may be justified. If reactions are positive, a course of immunotherapy will be recommended and may be of clinical value.

Geographic Distribution

For ease in finding allergenic trees of significance to individual practitioners, as well as the weeds and grasses discussed later in this chapter, clinically important species are listed on a region-by-region basis (Table 7–1). *Note that some states appear in more than one geographic region. In particular, states such as Florida, Texas, and California, which encompass large areas and widely diverse geophysical and climatic conditions, have more than one regional category.*

The sections listed are identified as follows:

United States: Most of the contiguous 48 states

Northeast: CT, MA, ME, MI, NH, NJ, NY, OH, PA, RI, VT

Middle Atlantic: DC, DE, MD, VA, WV

Southeast: AL, AR, FL, GA, KY, LA, MS, NC, SC, TN, east TX, VA

Midwest: CO, IA, IL, IN, KS, KY, MO, NB, ND, OK, SD

Intermountain: CO, ID, MT, ND, NV, OR, SD, UT, WA, WY

Southwest: AZ, CA, NM, NV, west TX

Texas: Central parts

Northwest: Northern CA, OR, WA

California: Central and southern parts

Allergenicity

The 1 to 4 numeric gradings assigned to pollen in the "Role in Allergy" column are measures of the relative importance of the particular pollen compared to others in the group. In general, the higher the number, the more allergenic the pollen. Other factors must also be considered, however. For example, a plant may produce pollen that is highly allergenic, yet so few plants may be present, or pollen production may be so sparse, that it really does not constitute a serious problem in clinical allergy. On the other hand, one plant's pollen may be moderately allergenic, but it may be so abundant that it causes a major problem. Therefore, when considering how important a plant is in allergy, one must consider both allergenicity and the amount of pollen produced.

This list is not a complete compilation of all allergenic species of trees. Many species have not been included because (1) only a few trees of a known allergenic species grow in a particular geographic area so there are not enough to constitute a problem; (2) their allergenicity has not yet been determined; (3) they are only potentially allergenic; or (4) have only a low order of allergenicity. Moreover, normal geographic habitats should not be interpreted too rigidly. The regional listings indicate the principal species naturally found in a specific locale; however, the desire to plant something different, or to introduce new and vigorous stock into the area, has spread nonindigenous species into new parts of the country

Furthermore, geographic borders are fuzzy and are not easily identified by the plants themselves. Except for species locked into specific borders, such as the saguaro cactus of the Sonoran Desert and the Joshua tree of the Mojave Desert, normal botanic distribution is not so easily defined. Therefore, even though the highest density of a particular plant may be found in the specific geographic locale given in Table 7–1, most plants continue to be found in decreasing concentrations as one moves out of the region. Even-

Table 7–1.   Major Regional Trees, Pollination Periods, and Allergic Potential

Predominant Genera	Botanical Group	Pollination Period	Role in Allergy*
ENTIRE UNITED STATES			
American elm	Elm	Feb.–Apr.	3
Chinese elm		Feb.–Apr.	3
Black walnut	Walnut	Apr.–May	2
Mulberry	Mulberry	Apr.–May	2
NORTHEAST			
Eastern red cedar	Cedar	Feb.–Apr.	2
Alder	Birch	Feb.–Mar.	3
Birch		Mar.–Apr.	3
Maple	Maple	Mar.–Apr.	3
Hickory	Hickory	May	3
American beech	Beech	May	2
Red oak		Apr.–May	4
White oak		May	4
American ash	Olive	Apr.–May	2
White poplar	Willow	Mar.–Apr.	3
Eastern sycamore	Plane tree	May	3
MIDDLE ATLANTIC			
Eastern red cedar	Cedar	Feb.–Apr.	2
Birch	Birch	Mar.–Apr.	3
Maple	Maple	Mar.–Apr.	3
Hickory	Hickory	May	3
American beech	Beech	May	2
Red oak		Apr.–May	4
White oak		May	4
American ash	Olive	Apr.–May	2
Black willow	Willow	Mar.–Apr.	2
White poplar		Mar.–Apr.	3
Eastern sycamore	Plane tree	May	3
SOUTHEAST AND SOUTH CENTRAL			
Eastern red cedar	Cedar	Feb.–Apr.	2
Virginia live oak	Beech	Mar.–Apr.	4
Red oak		Apr.–May	4
American ash	Olive	Apr.–May	2
Black willow	Willow	Mar.–Apr.	2
Pecan	Hickory	Mar.–Apr.	4
Eastern sycamore	Plane tree	May	3
SOUTHERN FLORIDA AND CARIBBEAN			
Cypress	Cedar	Mar.–Apr.	2
Australian pine	Misc.	Dec.–Jan.	3
MIDWEST			
Birch	Birch	Mar.–Apr.	3
Red oak	Beech	Apr.–May	4
White oak		May	4
Box elder	Maple	Mar.–Apr.	4
American ash	Olive	Apr.–May	2
Black willow	Willow	Mar.–Apr.	2
Cottonwood	Willow	Mar.–Apr.	3
CENTRAL TEXAS			
Mountain cedar	Cedar	Dec.–Feb.	4
Cedar elm	Elm	Sept.–Nov.	3
Virginia live oak	Beech	Mar.–Apr.	4
Scrub oak		Mar.–Apr.	4
Arizona ash	Olive	Mar.–Apr.	3
Olive		Feb.–Mar.	3
Black willow	Willow	Mar.–Apr.	2
Cottonwood		Mar.–Apr.	3
Eastern sycamore	Plane tree	May	3

Table 7–1.   Major Regional Trees, Pollination Periods, and Allergic Potential *Continued*

Predominant Genera	Botanical Group	Pollination Period	Role in Allergy*
INTERMOUNTAIN STATES			
Rocky mountain juniper	Juniper	Mar.–Apr.	2
Western juniper		Mar.–Apr.	2
Box elder	Maple	Mar.–Apr.	4
Cottonwood	Willow	Mar.–Apr.	3
Aspen		Mar.–May	3
SOUTHWEST			
Cypress	Cypress	Mar.–Apr.	2
Cedar elm	Elm	Sept.–Nov.	3
Pecan	Hickory	Mar.–Apr.	4
Scrub oak	Beech	Mar.–Apr.	4
Arizona ash	Olive	Apr.–May	3
Olive		Feb.–Mar.	3
Western sycamore	Plane tree	Mar.–May	3
English walnut	Walnut	Apr.–May	3
NORTHWEST			
Western juniper	Juniper	Mar.–Apr.	2
Alder	Birch	Feb.–Mar.	3
Hazelnut (filbert)	Birch	Feb.–Apr.	4
Box elder	Maple	Mar.–Apr.	4
Cottonwood	Willow	Mar.–Apr.	3
English walnut	Walnut	Apr.–May	3
Western sycamore	Plane tree	Mar.–May	3
SOUTHERN AND CENTRAL CALIFORNIA			
Cypress	Cedar	Mar.–Apr.	2
Alder	Birch	Feb.–Mar.	3
Hazelnut (filbert)		Feb.–Apr.	4
Coastal live oak	Beech	Mar.–Apr.	4
Olive	Olive	Feb.–Mar.	3
Western sycamore	Plane tree	Mar.–May	3
California black walnut	Walnut	Mar.–Apr.	3
English walnut		Apr.–May	3
Cottonwood	Willow	Mar.–Apr.	3
Australian pine	Misc.	Dec.–Jan.	3
Eucalyptus	Misc.	Feb.–Mar.	2

*1 to 4, in ascending order of allergenicity.

tually, climatic, geologic, or other factors ultimately preclude their continued growth and development.

Finally, pollination times for individual species also vary from region to region. Where the weather is warm throughout the year, or where warm weather returns early, pollination occurs at the early end of the pollination timespread. The farther north one goes, or the later warm weather returns, the later the onset of pollination. Yet in spite of the foregoing, tree pollination, for the most part, occurs between March and May, regardless of region or ambient temperature.

GRASSES (GRAMINEAE)

Compared to trees and weeds, few species of grasses exist. Pollination usually occurs from late spring to midsummer, although it may continue throughout the summer if weather conditions are proper and throughout the year in tropical and subtropical climates. Grass pollen is also found in fall pollen counts, but these pollens do not seem to be from the known allergenic species, and their allergenic significance is unknown. Individual species are difficult to identify by pollen morphology alone. Therefore, grass pollen counts usually identify the pollen only as grass, without naming the species.

Pollination

Normally, floral heads are formed when the shaft reaches a specific height. Grasses are survivors, however, and florets form even on closely cropped grass. This situation can present a more severe problem for dogs than for man because, as observed before, the tendency of dogs to walk with their noses to the ground, constantly sniffing, exposes them to a much larger potential antigen load than would ever be reached under other circumstances.

As with most aeroallergens, the time of day that pollen is released varies from species to species, although most release pollen during the early morning. This diurnal pattern may explain why some dogs that have spent a comfortable night sneeze or become pruritic after leaving the house in the morning.

Well-tended lawns can present another problem. As pets run through closely cropped grass, pollen may accumulate in their foot pads and between their toes, where the leaching action of sweat may release the antigenic components of the pollen and may cause a localized allergic reaction. Furthermore, some evidence suggests that the sap from cut grass may act as a contact allergen, or irritant, thereby creating additional problems as it accumulates on the feet.

Cross-Reactivity

The most cross-antigenic of the aeroallergens, grasses are the most likely to be suitable for testing and treatment as mixtures, rather than as individual antigens. Yet one should not use mixed antigens for allergy skin testing because, as discussed later, it is still possible to obtain negative reactions to grass mixtures in patients testing positive to individual grasses.

Allergenicity

Bermuda grass is probably the most allergenic species of grass in the United States. It is found throughout the southern half of the country and is slowly creeping northward. Its spread will no doubt be limited by climatic factors, although because of the temperate northwestern coastal climate, it grows almost as far north as British Columbia.

Most grasses not only are highly allergenic, but also have widespread distribution, as noted in Table 7–2.

As with trees, this listing is not all-inclusive, but contains species considered to be the most allergenically significant. Geo-

Table 7–2.   Major Regional Grasses, Pollination Periods, and Allergenic Potential

Botanical Group	Pollination Period	Role in Allergy*
LATE SPRING–EARLY SUMMER		
UNITED STATES		
Timothy		4
June (Bluegrass)		4
Fescue		3
Rye		4
NORTHEAST		
"Rye group"		
Orchard		3
Redtop		3
Sweet vernal		3
Velvet		3
MIDDLE ATLANTIC		
Bermuda		4
Johnson		3
"Rye group"		
Orchard		3
Redtop		3
Sweet vernal		3
SOUTHEAST		
Bermuda		4
Johnson		3
"Rye group"		
Sweet vernal		3
MIDWEST		
"Rye group"		
Orchard		3
Redtop		3
Brome		3
TEXAS		
"Rye group"		
Brome		3
Bermuda		4
Johnson		3
Bahia		3
INTERMOUNTAIN		
"Rye group"		
Brome		3
Bermuda		4
Johnson		3
CALIFORNIA AND SOUTHWEST		
Bahia		3
Bermuda		4
Johnson		3
Velvet		3
NORTHWEST		
Velvet		3

*1 to 4, in ascending order of allergenicity.

graphic distribution is also approximate, with some regional crossover and density variation, depending on the specific locale. For detailed information on local density and distribution, it is best to consult with local allergists, regional medical centers, and the technical service representatives of manufacturers of allergenic extracts.

WEEDS

Weeds constitute an extremely large and diverse group of plants. Allergenic weeds are found everywhere, with the number, variety, and density in any one location dependent on climate, altitude, and other geophysical conditions.

Sunflower Family (Compositae)

Compositae, or sunflower family, alone consists of about 15,000 species, but fortunately only a few are considered significant allergens. The most important allergenic weeds of this family are:

ragweeds	Genus ambrosia
marsh elders	Genus iva
cocklebur	Genus xanthium
sagebrushes, mugworts, and wormwoods	Genus artemisia

The principal source of antigen, of course, is pollen, although plant particles can also be allergenic. Studies with ragweed pollen and plant particles have shown that, when plants and pollen are wet, sufficient antigen can leach out to act as fine aerosol particles capable of eliciting a sensitivity response.[1] Skin tests with these aerosol particles have contained enough crude ragweed antigen and antigen E to elicit a positive reaction. Based on such studies, as well as observations of patients, weed pollen, or any other type of pollen or spores, can probably leach out antigen and cause reactions when pollen is trapped in the foot pads.

Genus Ambrosia

Probably the most significant allergenic weeds, at least in man, are the ambrosia, or ragweeds, which have probably about 40 or more species. Of these, the short and giant ragweed, found throughout the eastern and central United States and southeastern Canada, are the most important. Pollination, with some regional variation, usually begins in early August, reaches a peak about the first week in September, and continues well into October unless stopped by a killing frost.

Other species of ragweed, including the so-called "false ragweed" of the Far West, are found in other areas of the country, and their range and pollination times are listed in Table 7-3. Older texts may not show false ragweeds listed with the ambrosia or "true" ragweeds, because they were once thought to belong to other genera. They are now generally considered to belong to the ragweed group, although they still retain the false ragweed designation.

Genus Iva

Marsh elders have a wide distribution; some genera rival ragweed in pollen output and allergenicity. Rough marsh elder, in particular, which pollinates at about the same time as ragweeds, can add significantly to the allergenic load during that season.

Genus Xanthium

In spite of its universal distribution, cocklebur has a relatively low pollen output and is probably not a significant allergen, except under local conditions.

Genus Artemisia

The mugworts are significant allergens of the Northeast and Middle Atlantic states, as well as the Northwest. The other members of the genus are widely distributed from California, to the Great Lakes, to the Gulf states. A particularly heavy pollen producer is the annual sage, found in heavy concentration in Tennessee and its neighboring states.

Some insect-pollinated members of the composite family are cross-reactive with ragweed. These include goldenrod, marigolds, chrysanthemums, zinnias, dahlias, and asters, and although they are not generally responsible for pollinosis, they can cause clinical problems in ragweed-sensitive people when pollen concentrations are high or during close contact with the flower. As mentioned before, animals, with their propensity to stick their noses into flowers or onto pol-

Table 7–3. Major Regional Weeds, Pollination Times, and Allergic Potential

Predominant Genera	Botanical Group	Pollination Period	Role in Allergy*
ENTIRE UNITED STATES			
Cocklebur	Compositae	Sept.–Oct.	2
Lamb's-quarters	Chenopods	Aug.–Oct.	3
Rough pigweed	Amaranths	Aug.–Oct.	3
English plantain	Plantaginaceae	May–Sept.	3
NORTHEAST			
Short ragweed	Compositae	Aug.–Oct.	4
Tall ragweed			4
Mugwort			3
Sheep sorrel	Knotweed	May–July	1
Yellow dock			2
MIDDLE ATLANTIC			
Short ragweed	Compositae	Aug.–Oct.	4
Tall ragweed			4
Mugwort			4
Rough marsh elder			3
Sheep sorrel	Knotweed	May–July	1
Yellow dock			2
SOUTHEAST			
Short ragweed	Compositae	Aug.–Oct	4
Tall ragweed			4
Southern ragweed			3
Rough marsh elder			3
Dog fennel		Sept.–Nov.	2
Spiny pigweed	Amaranths	Sept.–Nov.	3
Sheep sorrel	Knotweed	May–July	1
Yellow dock			2
MIDWEST			
Short ragweed	Compositae	Aug.–Oct.	4
Tall ragweed			4
Burweed marsh elder			3
Sagebrush			3
Russian thistle	Chenopods	Aug.–Oct.	4
Kochia			4
Western water hemp	Amaranths	Aug.–Oct.	2
Yellow dock	Knotweed	May–July	2
TEXAS			
Short ragweed	Compositae	Aug.–Oct.	4
Tall ragweed			4
Western ragweed			3
Southern ragweed			3
Burweed marsh elder			3
Rough marsh elder			3
Dog fennel		Sept.–Nov.	2
Saltbush and scales	Chenopods	Aug.–Oct.	3
Russian thistle			4
Spiny pigweed	Amaranths	Aug.–Oct.	3
INTERMOUNTAIN			
Western ragweed	Compositae	Aug.–Oct.	3
False ragweed		June–Oct.	3
Sagebrush		Aug.–Oct.	3
Burweed marsh elder			3
Russian thistle	Chenopods	Aug.–Oct.	4
Kochia			4
Saltbush and scales			3

Table 7–3. Major Regional Weeds, Pollination Times, and Allergic Potential *Continued*

Predominant Genera	Botanical Group	Pollination Period	Role in Allergy*
NORTHWEST			
Sagebrush	Compositae	Aug.–Oct.	3
Mugwort			3
Saltbush and scales	Chenopods	Aug.–Oct.	3
SOUTHWEST			
Western ragweed	Compositae	Aug.–Oct.	3
False ragweed		June–Oct.	3
Sagebrush		Aug.–Oct.	3
Russian thistle	Chenopods	Aug.–Oct.	4
Kochia			4
Saltbush and scales			3
Spiny pigweed	Amaranths	Aug.–Oct.	3
CALIFORNIA			
False ragweed	Compositae	June–Oct.	3
Sagebrush		Aug.–Oct.	3
Saltbush and scales	Chenopods	Aug.–Oct.	3

*1 to 4, in ascending order of allergenicity.

len-laden ground, while sniffing lustily, are much more likely than man to receive a high enough dose to cause a reaction.

Goosefoot (Chenopodiaceae) and Carelessweed (Amaranthaceae) Families

Members of these families are closely related, with a similar pollen-grain structure and potential allergenicity. They are abundant, widely distributed, and prolific pollen producers. Fortunately, only a few species are clinically important.

Allergenically significant members of the goosefoot family include Russian thistle, which is really not a thistle but a tumbleweed, kochia, or burning bush, another tumbleweed, smotherweed, lamb's-quarters, saltbush, wingscale, greasewood, and sugar beet. Russian thistle and kochia are prolific pollen producers and highly allergenic, with Russian thistle rivaling, and even exceeding, the importance of ragweed as an allergen in some areas. Sugar beet is extremely prolific and allergenic when cultivated for seed production, whereas lamb's-quarters may be the least important allergen of this group.

Carelessweed, another large group, has several members that produce extremely high numbers of allergenic pollen. The most important members of this family are Palmer's amaranth, western water hemp, pigweed, and spiny amaranth.

Hemp Family (Cannabinaceae)

The only known allergenically important pollen in this group is hemp. Other members, such as nettles and hops, are prolific pollen producers, but their allergenicity is uncertain.

Plantain Family (Plantaginaceae)

English plantain is the only member of this family considered a significant allergen. It has a long pollination season, reaching a peak in June and July; however, pollination can start as early as May and may continue into the fall. Fortunately, pollen production is scant for the most part, and except in the Pacific Northwest and pockets of local density, atmospheric pollen is insufficient to cause serious problems by itself.

Knotweed Family (Polygonaceae)

Sheep sorrel (red sorrel) is the only allergenically important pollen producer in this group. The sorrels are widely distributed throughout North America and are heavy pollen producers. Geographic location and approximate pollination times are found in Table 7–3.

Distribution and Allergenicity

Many weeds have a wide geographic distribution; some plants are found throughout the United States. As with trees and grasses,

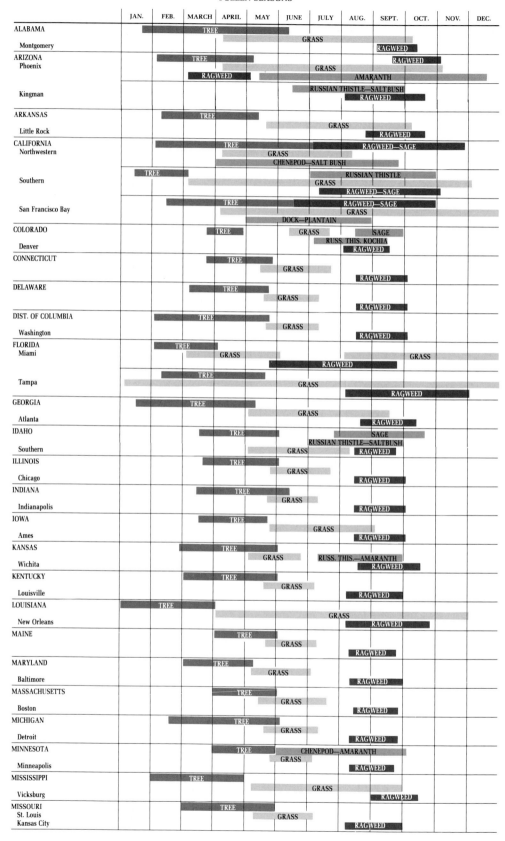

Fig. 7–1. Pollen seasons in the continental United States. (From Feinberg, S.: Allergy in Practice. Chicago, Year Book, 1944.)

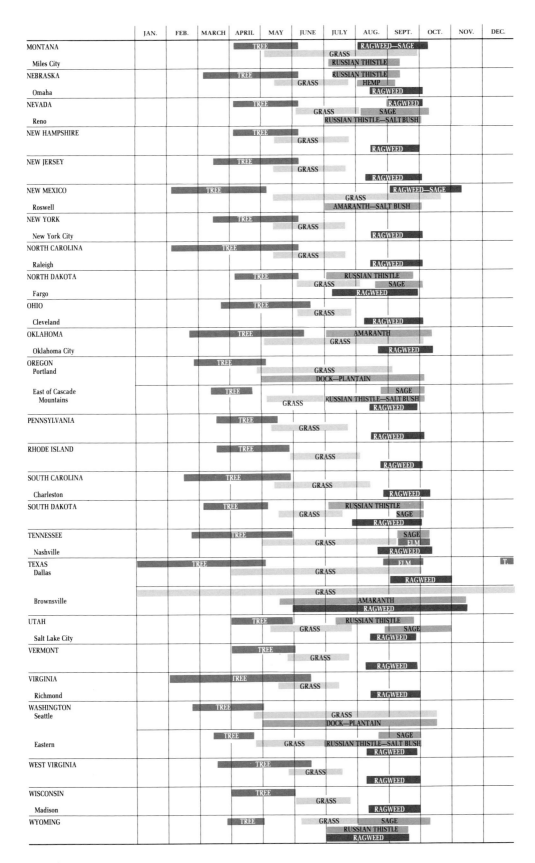

Fig. 7–1. *Continued.*

the pollination times (listed in Table 7–3) are approximate, with the actual onset and completion of pollination dependent on such climatic conditions as local temperatures, onset of warm weather, time of the first frost, and the amount of rain and heat during the growing season.

Weed pollens, as previously noted, are not homogeneous, but are generally complex structures containing multiple allergens of varying significance. Short ragweed, for example, contains over 50 allergens, of which the most significant in man are antigens E and K. Although these are probably the important antigens in animals as well, until specific research has definitively shown their significance, it will have to remain an assumption.

To add to their allergenic potential, some weeds are also prolific pollen producers, depending on species and climatic conditions during the growing season. For example, one ragweed plant alone can produce up to one billion pollen grains during the pollination period. Multiplied by the millions of possible ragweed plants in any geographic area, this represents a tremendous potential for severe reaction and discomfort.

The time of day of pollen release and distribution also vary from species to species, but most plants release their pollen during the morning. Its distribution depends on the temperature and the amount of wind; pollen travels farther on warm updrafts or windy days than in a cooler, still atmosphere. Rain also plays a role by washing pollen out of the air and reducing thereby the pollen load.

Finally, cross-allergenicity, which can be seen among closely related species of weeds, not only increases the severity of an allergic attack, but also is a consideration when one evaluates patients new to a specific geographic locale. Although the patient may not have been previously exposed to a specific plant, an individual may still react because of sensitivity to a closely related, cross-reactive species.

To keep the pollination times for weeds, trees, and grasses in perspective, Figure 7–1 is a state-by-state calendar of their approximate pollination dates.

MOLDS

Many veterinary dermatologists regard allergy to molds as a relatively insignificant clinical problem. This attitude is archaic, but understandable, because many physicians ascribed little allergenic importance to molds until recent years. Because the practitioner must rely on specialists for information and guidance, however, the unfortunate consequence is that he may not fully appreciate the significance of these universally distributed and highly allergenic particles.

Historical Perspectives

Unlike pollen allergy, the first suspected case of mold or fungal allergy was not described until 1930, in a human patient with eczema and asthma. The diagnostic workup was incomplete, however, so one cannot say with absolute assurance that the problem was due to molds. The first definitively reported case was in 1935, and since then a vast literature has evolved to prove the importance of mold allergy in man.

Mold allergy is no less important in lower animals, although its relative significance varies from species to species. Dogs, for example, are in a high-clinical-incidence category, based on my own observations and clinical studies during the past 30 years. Studies on inhalant allergies in cats are still in the early investigative stage, and therefore, one cannot make an absolute statement on the significance of molds in cats at this time. Heaves, caused by moldy hay, is a good example of apparent mold sensitivity in the horse, and fog fever is apparently caused by a reaction to molds in cattle.

My own interest in mold sensitivity began over 30 years ago with a dog that I was treating for seasonal pollinosis. At the time, I was only testing for a few environmental agents and a representative sampling of tree, grass, and weed pollens. I was unaware of the importance of molds in inhalant allergy at that time. The dog had responded well to immunotherapy and was comfortable as long as he stayed near his home in northern New Jersey. Whenever he was taken to Cape Cod by the family for their summer vacation, however, his condition deteriorated dramatically.

Being a novice at the time, I wrote to a physician allergist in Cape Cod and inquired about allergens that were important in that area or were different from those that I might find locally. He was kind enough to respond that the common allergens were similar in both locations, but Cape Cod had a high density of molds, particularly mucor, fusarium, and rhizopus.

The dog was skin tested, found positive to two of the three molds, and given immunotherapy. To my gratification, the response was excellent, and the final result was a comfortable patient, a satisfied client, and a newly aware veterinarian.

Sensitivity to molds helps to explain the presence of allergic signs at times other than the ordinarily accepted and recognized allergy seasons. Although one may think of seasonally recurrent allergy as falling into neat little time slots, coinciding with the onset and completion of various pollen seasons, a patient's history often indicates severe problems long before the first pollen grain is released and well after the last pollen has left the atmosphere for the season. In fact, in the northern snow belt area, clinical signs often continue until a sustained hard frost or until snow covers the ground. During winter thaws or sudden warm spells, clinical signs often recur.

Because no plants are pollinating at that time, it is unlikely that anything other than molds that have been suddenly stirred up after lying dormant on the frozen or snow-covered ground can be responsible for the problem. Furthermore, in suddenly pruritic dogs that have already undergone immunotherapy to molds, a single booster injection of the mold allergens without other treatment is often enough to reverse clinical signs and return the dog to normal.

Biologic Considerations

It has been aptly said that we live in a moldy world, rather than a world with molds. To appreciate the magnitude of the situation, we have no accurate figures for the total number of mold species, but estimates vary from 100,000 to 250,000 individual species. In addition, molds can be prolific spore formers. One species of mushroom alone, during its 6-day sporulation period, produces **60 million spores per hour, 24 hours a day.** Multiply this figure by 6 days and we have a figure that is impossible to comprehend, and that is for just one mushroom.

Now consider the number of fungal species and the number of individuals making up the species, and it is easy to understand the potential magnitude of mold allergy. Fortunately, only about a dozen species are considered significant sensitizers, and perhaps an equal number are moderately allergenic. Thus, out of the mass of mold species, only a minuscule number are potentially clinically significant.

Fungi have a worldwide distribution and occur over every land mass. Only the atmosphere over large bodies of water may be free of fungi. Although the word "fungus" is abhorrent to most people, life as we know it would not continue without them. Not only are fungi integral to the decomposition and disintegration of dead organic matter, but also they play a vital role in daily life. They supply us with edible mushrooms, as well as fermenting grain and fruit for beer and wine production. In the form of brewer's yeast, fungi are an important source of B vitamins; moreover, the baking industry could not exist without them. In addition, many other edible species of fungus produce cheese and add interest and variety to everyday meals. Mold-sensitive patients should avoid eating yeasty, fermented, or moldy foods because these can provoke both gastrointestinal and pruritic clinical signs in such individuals. It is also conceivable that dry pet foods that are not fresh, or are stored improperly, may support mold growth and may thereby precipitate an allergic attack in mold-sensitive animals.

Although most fungi are saprophytic, living on dead or decaying vegetation, a few are parasitic, thrive on live tissue, and cause disease. They are members of the plant family, with well-defined cell walls and prominent nuclei, but no chlorophyll. Molds may be unicellular or multicellular with branching hyphae, which may or may not have septa. Whereas the terms hypha and hyphae refer to the individual filaments, they are called the mycelium when considered as a whole.

Molds have a wide growth and survival

range, from altitudes below sea level to high, mountainous areas. They can survive in temperatures ranging from about 160°F to sub-freezing, but they grow most luxuriantly in tropical and subtropical climates and during warm months in more temperate regions. Wet or humid weather is conducive to growth in most species, and it also stimulates sporulation in many varieties. Spores are much lighter than pollen and can float for long periods of time, allowing them to be dispersed over much wider areas than pollen. Although some species reach their highest spore concentrations during light, warm periods, most settle much more densely in the cooler evening temperature. Therefore, mold-sensitive patients are frequently much more symptomatic at night than during the day.

Molds may be classified structurally or by mode of reproduction. As with many plants, reproduction may be sexual or asexual. Morphologically, fungi fall into two broad structural groups: yeasts and hyphal forms. Yeasts are predominantly unicellular organisms that reproduce by budding or fission. Some new cells split off completely, whereas others form long chains or buds. Some yeasts also have a mycelial phase, depending on growth conditions and culture media. One of the culturally identifiable characteristics of Candida albicans, for example, is its ability to form hyphae in proper culture media.

Although spores are probably the most antigenic portion of the mold, any structural element is potentially allergenic, including cell-wall fragments, hyphae, and yeast cell bodies. Mold spore concentrations are usually seasonal, but seasons are not as clear-cut as with many pollens. Soil contains high concentrations of mold spores that lie dormant while the ground is frozen or covered with snow. At the first thaw, and particularly when ground cover is sparse, every gust of wind stirs up the spores or other fungal elements, which suddenly appear in the atmosphere in sufficient concentration to cause problems in mold-sensitive individuals.

Therefore, in areas with a definite winter season, molds first peak in late February or early March, with a second peak frequently seen in mid- to late July. Whether this summer peak reflects the hot, humid weather usual at this time or whether it is due to other factors is uncertain. A third peak occurs from late October until December, owing to the large amounts of dead or decaying leaves and dead grass lying on the ground. This peak continues until the ground is frozen or adequately covered with snow.

Distribution

Fungi have a universal distribution, being found over every land mass in the world. By far, the largest number are the extramural or outdoor molds, whereas the intramural or indoor molds are a much smaller group. One should not then assume that the two categories are sharply divided because crossover is common, and many species occur in both classes. Their predominant location in nature therefore determines their classification.

At no time is the atmosphere totally free of molds, so depending on climatic conditions, spores or particles are always found to a greater or lesser extent in the air. When the ground is frozen or covered with snow, spore counts are low, rising to high concentrations as the ground thaws, the temperature rises, atmospheric moisture increases, or other conditions for mold growth and distribution improve.

As mentioned previously, dead or decaying vegetation is an excellent substrate for mold growth, although molds can attack and parasitize living vegetation, as occurs with rusts and smuts. Mulch piles, compost heaps, and leaf piles are virtual mold generators, producing spores and particles by the billions. Shrubbery beds, because of the rich organic nature of the soil, are also ideal breeding grounds for molds. Therefore, dogs living in suburban areas and digging in shrubbery beds or running through leaf piles in the fall have a greater risk of developing clinical signs than dogs living in more urban environments.

Lest one think that the small number of indoor species makes them unimportant, their distribution and ease of growth put these molds into a high-allergenic-risk category. Indoor molds can be so prevalent that some allergists consider them a major component of house dust and equal in importance to the house dust mite in the initiation of an allergic attack. The ability of molds to thrive on almost any substrate, as long as they have a source of carbon and moisture, with a few essential elements, makes them particularly difficult to control.

Clinical Significance

The wholesale distribution of molds and their tenacity of growth present serious problems for the allergic patient. Even foam rubber pillows, in spite of their reputation as a hypoallergenic material, support mold growth. More common sources of indoor molds include refrigerator drip pans and evaporator coils, refrigerator door gaskets, water pipes, sink cabinets, and dishwasher doors. Most foods provide excellent substrates for molds, which grow well on fruit and melon rinds, peels and outer vegetable leaves, dairy products, and meat. Molds are found in beer, wine, pickled foods, and many cheeses and may cause clinical problems in sensitive individuals.

Molds also thrive in damp basements and musty attics, air-conditioner and other filters, humidifiers, rug padding, old wallpaper and paste, masonry, and almost any imaginable environmental condition.

Allergenic species of molds have also been cultured from seborrheic and other lesions involving the skin and coat. These molds probably contribute minimally to the patient's ambient allergen load, but they may cause pruritus by a direct action of spores or hyphal elements on the skin.

Thus, it is easy to see that molds represent a much more significant source of allergens than previously considered. Furthermore, their diversity, universal distribution, and tremendous capacity for spore formation create a serious potential for causing both seasonal and nonseasonal problems. Therefore, molds must be suspected in all allergic reactions either occurring out of the normal allergy seasons or not responding to specific immunotherapy for other inhalant or environmental allergens. Consequently, all known indigenous allergenic molds should be included in any skin-testing program.

Taxonomic Classification

The terms fungus and mold are commonly used interchangeably in allergy, regardless of species or type. Although the taxonomic classification of these species makes interesting reading, such a classification is not essential to the diagnosis and treatment of mold allergy and is only discussed briefly.

The four major fungal groups of allergenic interest are the Zygomycetes, Ascomycetes, Basidiomycetes and the Fungi Imperfecti. These can be further divided into several subgroups based on taxonomy, cultural characteristics, and reproduction.

Zygomycetes

The Zygomycetes comprise a small group, producing a sexual resting cell or zygospore, from which the group takes its name. The principal allergenic genera in this class are rhizopus and mucor.

Ascomycetes

The common bond of the Ascomycetes, which contain the largest number of species, is the presence of an ascus, or sac, to carry the sexual spores. This group is composed of both yeasts and hyphal forms, most of which are soil saprophytes. Plant and animal disease agents are also found in this group, however. Ascomycetes contain such delicacies as morels and truffles, as well as the allergenic species of chaetomium.

Basidiomycetes

The common feature of the Basidiomycetes is a basidium, or club-like structure. The basidiospores are attached to the basidia by fine hyphal structures from which they are detached and disseminated by wind currents. Under proper stimulation, some basidiospores eject their spores like shot, and these are referred to as ballistospores. The Basidiomycetes are among the most prolific of the fungal spore producers, but except for rusts and smuts, their allergenicity has not been studied thoroughly. Considering the potentially high density of basidiospores in the atmosphere, one may assume that additional allergenic species will be found, when studied.

Fungi Imperfecti

The final group is the asexual fungi, or Fungi Imperfecti. Taxonomically, no structural features link these fungi together, except the lack of sexual apparatus. Some sources refer to this group as the form class Deuteromycetes. Many important fungal allergens are found in this group, which includes botrytis, fusarium, alternaria, helminthosporium, geotrichum, penicillium, aspergillus, torulopsis, candida, and rhodotorula.

Classification by Location

From the allergist's point of view, it can be helpful to think of molds in terms of whether they are primarily extramural, intramural, or both. These classifications are not absolutes because the distinctions are often blurred, and some molds belong to both categories. The classification, therefore, really refers to the mold's principal habitat. Because many molds share common habitats and occur in equally high concentrations both indoors and out, they may be properly placed in a mixed category. Regardless of their principal habitat, however, when spore concentrations are high enough, they are often found everywhere.

Moreover, fungi that normally grow in soil or organic debris can also be found in the soil of potted plants. Therefore, although soil molds are classified as outdoor molds, they could reasonably be considered as both indoor and outdoor varieties.

Outdoor Molds

The principal outdoor molds of allergenic interest are as follows:

1. **ALTERNARIA** is an abundant species found throughout the country, although uncommon in the Northwest. It is chiefly a plant parasite.

2. **CLADOSPORIUM (HORMODENDRUM), EPICOCCUM, TORULOPSIS,** and **RHODOTORULA** grow on dead and decaying vegetation and have an abundant, universal distribution.

3. **CANDIDA** has a widespread distribution on plants and is occasionally found in high enough concentration to be an aeroallergen. Under proper conditions, it can also colonize and become infectious to animal tissue.

4. **AUREOBASIDIUM PULLULANS (PULLULARIA PULLULANS),** another allergen with a wide distribution, commonly occurs in both soil and on vegetation. It can deteriorate both plastic and painted surfaces, especially in hot and humid climates.

5. **GEOTRICHUM,** as its name suggests, is frequently found in soil and is a common contaminant of dairy products.

6. **TRICHODERMA,** found in damp soil and rotting timber, is widely distributed over large parts of the country.

7. **RUSTS, SMUTS,** and **MILDEWS** are important plant parasites with a widespread distribution in nature. Rusts attack many types of crop and ornamental plants, whereas smuts are a particularly important parasite of many cereal grains. The powdery mildews are parasitic for a wide variety of plants; the downy mildews are commonly found on grasses, grapes, onions, and other cultivated crops.

8. **EPIDERMOPHYTON** and **TRICHOPHYTON** are soil contaminants and, in high enough concentration, may be responsible for allergic reactions. Trichophyton may also parasitize animal tissue.

9. **STEMPHYLIUM** parasitizes the leaves and stems of vegetable crops, and its spores are commonly released into the air during the daytime.

10. **CURVULARIA** is a common parasite of grasses. Normally, the concentration of spores is highest in the early afternoon, but mowing can easily disperse spores at any time.

11. **DRECHSLERA SAROKINIANA (HELMINTHOSPORIUM SATIVUM)** is also a common allergenic parasite of grasses and cereal grains. As with curvularia, the concentration of this mold is normally highest in the early afternoon. Here, too, grain-threshing operations can release large quantities of spores into the air at any time.

12. **NIGROSPORA,** named for its black spores, grows saprophytically on organic debris in the soil. Each day during its growing season, its spores are propelled into the air like cannon shot between 11 A.M. and 1 P.M.

Indoor Molds

The principal indoor molds of allergenic interest are as follows:

1. **MUCOR** and **RHIZOPUS** are primarily indoor molds, but they commonly occur in outdoor air samples, as well.

2. **NEUROSPORA INTERMEDIA (MONILIA SITOPHILA),** the "red bread mold," is common in bakeries and flour mills. Uncontaminated outdoor air is usually free of this mold.

3. **PENICILLIUM** species constitute a large genus very commonly found in indoor air. These molds contaminate food and other organic matter and are also used commercially in food and antibiotic production.

4. **SCOPULARIOPSIS** commonly occurs on meat and cheese, as well as on many types of decaying organic matter.

5. **ASPERGILLUS** species are common, universal indoor molds.

Mixed Indoor and Outdoor Molds

Among the molds found both indoors and outdoors are the following:

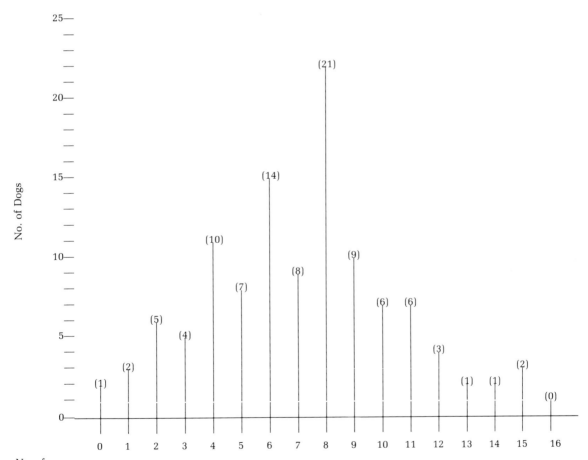

Fig. 7–2.   Positive mold reactions in a review of 100 allergic dogs. The average number of reactions per dog was 6.6 (median = 5).

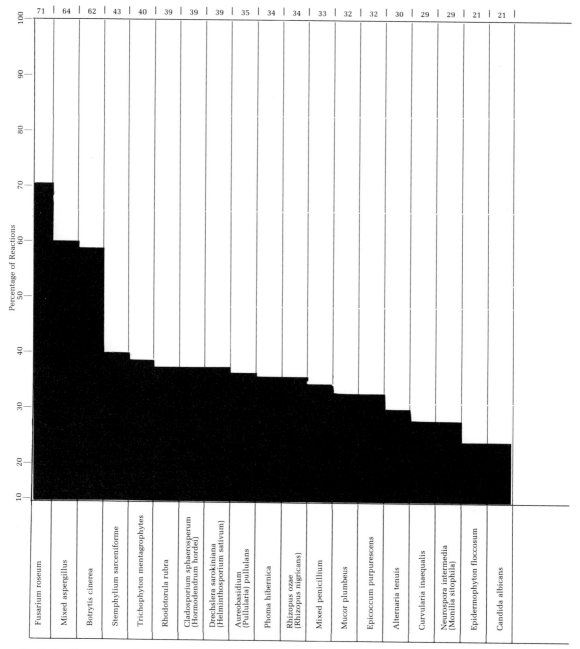

| | 71 | 64 | 62 | 43 | 40 | 39 | 39 | 39 | 35 | 34 | 34 | 33 | 32 | 32 | 30 | 29 | 29 | 21 | 21 | |

Fig. 7–3.   Percentage of positive mold reactions found in a survey of 100 allergic dogs.

1. Yeasts and yeast-like organisms, such as **SACCHAROMYCES ACTINOMYCES,** are commonly found in orchards, dairies, and breweries.

2. **BOTRYTIS** is a widely distributed, common plant pathogen found throughout the year.

3. **CHAETOMIUM** is commonly found in warm, humid areas, on damp straw, manure, pasteboard, and textiles.

4. **FUSARIUM** species are parasitic on veg-

etable and field crops; however, they also can occur on stored fruits and vegetables, a feature that gives them a widespread distribution.

The foregoing are by no means complete or exhaustive lists of mold allergens, nor are all listed molds equally allergenic. Although some mold genera have a universal distribution, species and concentrations differ because of climatic, environmental, and geographic location. Moreover, as additional clinical case studies are conducted, species now considered nonallergenic, or of minimal allergenic importance, will doubtless be added to the list of allergens.[2]

Cross-Reactivity and Relative Allergenicity

Finally little cross-reactivity exists among molds, with the exception of alternaria, Drechslera sarokiniana (Helminthosporium sativum) stemphylium, and curvularia, which seem to show some cross-antigenicity. Therefore, for testing and treatment, mixed molds should be avoided, and only individual molds should be used.

To evaluate the relative significance of different molds in my patients, I made a retrospective review of positive mold reactions in 100 consecutive dogs (Figs. 7–2 and 7–3). As can be seen, the highest numbers of reactions were obtained against Fusarium roseum, mixed aspergillus species, and Botrytis cinerea, with the smallest percentage against Candida albicans. The number of reactions per dog ranged from 0 for 1 dog to 15 for 2 dogs, whereas the average number of reactions per dog was 6.66, and the median number was 5.

REFERENCES

1. Solomon, W.R.: Uncovering the "fine details" of pollen allergen transport. J. Allergy Clin. Immunol., *74*:674, 1984.
2. Caplin, I., and Haynes, J.T.: Mold allergy. Ann. Allergy, *28*:87, 1970.

Environmental Allergens

Environmental allergens are a widely diverse group, varying from household to household and region to region. Variation depends on such factors as life styles, furniture, floor and wall coverings, clothing fabrics, and hobbies. As examples, woodworking hobbyists have wood dusts not found in the average household; metalworkers have metal particles, cutting oils, and other materials needed by the machinist and metalworker; potters have clay dusts and colors; artists and their families are exposed to canvas, oils, water colors, and solvents. All these factors must be considered when taking the patient's medical history. Dedicated allergists have even been known to visit the homes of their unresponsive patients, to ensure that nothing has been overlooked in the patient's history.

Some environmental allergens discussed here have not yet been incriminated in animal allergy. Because they are either known or highly suspect sensitizers in man, however, it is likely that, as with other allergens, sensitivity will eventually be demonstrated in the dog. At the least, the reader will become "sensitized" to the problem and will have a better chance of recognizing it, should it occur.

HOUSE DUST AND ITS COMPONENTS AND HOUSEHOLD INSECT ALLERGENS

House Dust and Dust Mites

House dust is probably the most common environmental allergen and perhaps the most troublesome. It is considered by some to be truly a witch's brew, with no two dusts identical. In all probability it contains molds, household plant particles, fabric particles from rugs, padding, draperies, and even clothing, paper particles, tobacco smoke, particles brought or blown in from the outside, particles circulated from the heating or cooling systems, and other particles indigenous to the particular household.

Commercially prepared dust extract is gathered from representative dust sources, extracted, filtered, and concentrated. It is then standardized and rediluted into standard market concentrations.[1] Although commercial dust extracts are fairly representative of dust in general, individual households may contain allergens indigenous only to that household. If the patient's medical history and allergy skin testing substantiate a diagnosis of dust allergy, but the patient fails to respond adequately to house dust immunotherapy, it may be necessary to prepare an autogenous dust from the patient's household in order to effect a positive therapeutic result.

Although dust is present throughout the year, dust load increases seasonally in many parts of the country, particularly when hot-air heating systems or air conditioners are first turned on. Even steam or hot-water heating systems can increase dust exposure in a room through warm-air convection currents. These currents carry dust particles with them as the warm air rises, only to have them drop again as the air cools near the ceiling, thus bringing dust particles into closer contact with the patient. Because dogs and cats are at floor level, where the concentration is highest, they have an even greater potential exposure than man.

The house dust mite has received much attention in the human literature in recent years and, in fact, is considered by many investigators to be the principal allergenic component of house dust (Fig. 8–1). Most mites are members of the Dermatophagoides species and have a worldwide distribution.

Dust mites thrive in warm, damp environments and live in pillows, mattresses, carpets, or any other material containing human scale and dander, on which they feed. In cooler, drier weather, their body fragments and fecal particles become airborne, increas-

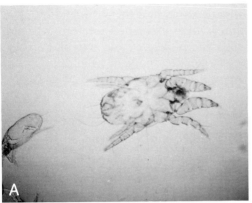 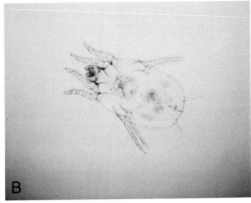

Fig. 8–1. House dust mites. *A,* Dermatophagoides farinae (male, ventral view). *B,* D. pteronyssinus (male, ventral view). (Courtesy of Greer Laboratories, Lenoir, NC.)

ing allergen load and exposure. Cross-reactivity with other mite species has not been studied extensively, and until such studies are done, one must consider the possibility that exposure to parasitic mites could cause a positive reaction to dust mites. In fact, one recent study suggests a cross-reaction with ear mites. Until more studies are done, however, and without evidence to the contrary, a positive skin-test reaction to dust mite must be evaluated in the same light as any other positive test.

Sawdust and Wood Dust

Sawdust and wood dust can be important sensitizers, especially in houses where woodworking is done as a hobby and in houses undergoing renovation that requires extensive carpentry work, with its resultant dust. If a pet has a nonseasonal allergic problem, and if the type of wood that is producing the dust is known, one may often obtain test antigens to the specific wood to determine whether a sensitivity to the particular dust actually exists. Immunotherapy is of limited value in these cases, and the best treatment is to keep the pet out of the rooms where the dusts are generated, to keep the area as well ventilated as possible, and, if the house has a forced-air heating system or central air conditioning, to ensure that the filters are kept scrupulously clean.

Metalworking Dust

Allergic reactions associated with metalworking are invariably of the delayed-hyper-sensitivity type; inhalant reactions, such as seen with organic dusts, are rare. On the other hand, frequent or prolonged contact with certain metals, such as chrome or nickel, can cause contact-allergic reactions involving the skin, as discussed in more detail in Chapter 14. In addition, machine cutting oils are a potential problem for machinists and their pets. For example, I once treated a cat that was presented with an apruritic dermatosis in which the superficial epidermis of the legs had peeled off as though sliced with a dermatome. The underlying skin was satiny smooth, with no evidence of inflammation. The cat belonged to a metal hobbyist and was in the habit of walking over the workbench, then licking the cutting oil off its feet. Whether this represents an idiosyncratic or toxicity reaction is uncertain, but 2 months after the cat had been banished from the workroom, he again had a full coat with no further evidence of sloughing skin.

Tobacco Dust and Smoke

Tobacco dust and smoke is generally considered an irritant, rather than an allergen, and the significance of positive skin-test reactions is uncertain. In man, tobacco smoke can initiate or exacerbate an asthmatic attack, probably because of its irritating qualities. I have also seen dogs begin to sneeze and tear when exposed to tobacco smoke. Whether this is due to allergy or irritation is open to question. Nevertheless, if a reaction occurs in a patient following exposure to tobacco smoke, one should make every effort to avoid contact with smoke in that patient.

Cockroach Antigens

We have known for some time that inhaled cockroach antigens, derived from distintegrating body parts or fecal matter, can produce allergic reactions in man. The degree to which this can become a problem depends on climatic conditions and household sanitation. In warm, humid climates, and particularly in apartment houses where cockroaches can move freely from apartment to apartment along water pipes and other common communicating structures, these insects can be difficult to control. The higher the cockroach population, with its attendant increase in available atmospheric antigens, the more likely the tendency to develop an allergy.

To date, cockroach sensitivity has not been reported in the dog or cat. I have been testing dogs with cockroach antigen experimentally for 1 year and find only an occasional positive reaction. Whether this indicates that the dog is not especially sensitive to the cockroach antigens or that my patients come from an environmentally select population will not be answered until other veterinary allergists, in different parts of the country, test a sufficiently diverse population of dogs to draw a conclusion.

Environmental Pollutants

Dogs have been used as experimental models in the study of the harmful effects of environmental pollutants, but the role of these noxious substances as sensitizers or allergens for dogs and cats is speculative at this time. Unlike in man, in whom allergic and respiratory problems are directly and definitively associated with poor air quality, such problems have not been adequately reported in the veterinary literature.

Food Odors

Food odors are occasional causes of allergic asthma and allergic eczema in man. Because odors are actually minute particles in an aerosol suspension, it is not unreasonable to assume that dogs and cats with a known food allergy could occasionally develop an allergic reaction if the particulate concentration is high enough. Therefore, one should keep food-allergic pets out of the kitchen when cooking foods to which they are allergic, unless the kitchen is well ventilated or cooking is done under a hood with a strong exhaust fan.

Newspaper and Newsprint

Newspaper and newsprint cause immediate and delayed hypersensitivity problems in occasional pets. Probably, no single agent in the ink or paper is responsible for the allergic reactions because they may be due to dust, paper mites, ink, and aniline dyes. Paper mites live on old paper and probably cause allergic reactions in much the same way as the dust mites; they may, in fact, be cross-reactive with the house dust mite. Molds also live on old paper and contribute to their decomposition. Allergic reactions could occur following exposure to both mold and degenerating paper particles. Ink and dyes, on the other hand, are more likely to cause contact sensitivity, especially if the paper becomes wet when used as a cage or bed liner.

If a nonresponsive allergy exists, and if the pet spends much time on newspaper, the best course of action would be to remove the paper from the immediate environment and to evaluate the patient's response. A positive allergy skin test for newsprint helps to confirm the diagnosis, but a negative response does not rule it out.

Caterpillar Droppings

A possible new, and heretofore unreported, source of allergens for pets may be caterpillar or other insect droppings. During the summer of 1989, I treated two dogs that I suspect may be allergic to these droppings. Both dogs had allergies that were under excellent control following treatment for other inhalants, only to become suddenly extremely pruritic and unresponsive to booster allergy injections.

Both clients observed and reported a locally heavy infestation of gypsy moth caterpillars; droppings were everywhere, covering walks, lawns, and porches. Avoidance was impossible, so exposure was constant until the caterpillars pupated and the droppings were removed by the elements. The severity of clinical signs seemed to coincide with the appearance of the droppings and then to improve as the droppings disappeared. On reflection, one client recalled that a similar situation had occurred the previous year.

A crude extract was made from caterpillar droppings, and one dog was tested intradermally with a 10-fold dilution and a 100-fold dilution. Positive skin-test reactions were obtained to both dilutions. Whether this represents a true clinical sensitivity or a nonspecific reaction, is still purely speculative.*

No definite evidence, as yet, has incriminated the gypsy moth, inchworm, or other caterpillar in allergy, but the proteinaceous quality of their droppings and the probability that these droppings will disintegrate into fine particles and disperse in the atmosphere make them likely environmental allergens. A report in the human literature has also suggested insect dropping and other particulate sensitivity among entomologists.

PLANTS AND FIBERS

Kapok

Kapok, derived from the kapok tree, is an important plant fiber sensitizer. Its soft, fluffy fibers are commonly found in throw pillows, stuffed toys, and older upholstered furniture. Interestingly, kapok as well as cotton and some other fibers are not allergenic when fresh, but as they age and deteriorate, chemical changes that apparently occur in the fibers render the material allergenic.

Cotton Linters

Cotton linters are short fibers that adhere to the cottonseed when the long fibers have been removed by the gin. These fibers are used to make absorbent cotton, wadding, carpets, felt, and twine, as well as to stuff mattresses, throw pillows, and upholstered furniture. As these fibers age, they too begin to change and deteriorate, releasing miroscopic particles into the air that may be allergenic.

Cotton fabric made from long-staple fibers

is generally not considered allergenic and is usually accepted as safe to sleep on. If the fabric is made of yarn in which the short, linter fibers have been incorporated with the long staples, however, it may become allergenic.

Cottonseed

Cottonseed is a potentially important allergen in two respects. First, the water-soluble fraction is a potent sensitizer, but one more likely to be encountered in processing plants than under normal household conditions. Second, cottonseed meal is a frequent component of livestock feed, as well as some pet foods, and can cause both inhalant and ingestant allergies.

Pyrethrum

Pyrethrum is an insecticide derived from the dried flowers of the chrysanthemum plant, a member of the composite family, and can be both an allergen and an irritant. Allergic reactions are not common, but pets allergic to ragweed or other members of the composite family are more likely to be sensitive to pyrethrum. Although sensitivity can develop to any available form of the insecticide, it is most likely to develop against the powder because it lies in the animal's coat as loose particulate matter and is more likely to be inhaled over a long period than are dips or sprays.

ANIMAL HAIR AND DANDER

Wool

Wool has led a precarious existence as an allergen; many allergists consider it important, whereas others consider it only a minor allergen, or even only an irritant. Microscopically, wool fibers are sharp and barbed, supporting the theory of irritant potential. Under any circumstances, older wool blankets, rugs, and garments are more likely to be a problem than new ones because older fibers begin to fragment and break up into minute particles.

Feathers

Feathers seem to be an important group of animal allergens. Although statistical eval-

*For personal reference. This information is not published, but was presented as an abstract at the Aspen Allergy Conference in July, 1988.

uations have not been made and definitive data are not available, this opinion is based on two factors: (1) allergic dogs that sleep on feather pillows and mattresses often improve dramatically when the bedding is changed to inert materials; and (2) these dogs, as well as others, often have positive skin-test reactions to feathers. Here, too, feathers are apparently not particularly allergenic when fresh, but they become increasingly problematic as they age, so old pillows, down comforters, vests, and mattresses can become a significant source of allergens. Pet birds within the household, or heavy concentrations of pigeons, crows, or other birds in the general environment, can also present a problem. The allergenic potential for proteins in bird droppings on lawns and in fields where dogs run is high, especially as the droppings begin to dry and particles become airborne. No information available at this time indicates whether this presents a real problem for dogs and cats, however.

Cross-allergenicity among different species of feathers seems to be strong, so extracts for both testing and treatment generally consist of mixtures of chicken, duck, and goose feathers. When feather allergy exists, it is best not to keep pet birds; if birds must be kept, one must keep the cages scrupulously clean, not allow feathers or droppings to accumulate, and keep the allergic dog or cat out of the room where the birds are kept. Outdoors, one should keep pets away from areas where birds congregate and away from their droppings.

Animal Danders

Animal danders, particularly dog, cat, and human, have occasionally caused positive skin-test reactions in animals and been presumed responsible for some cases of clinical allergy. Admittedly, this is difficult to prove because dogs rarely have positive reactions to single allergens. Yet I have seen clinical improvement in dogs that tested positive to other dogs or cats when these patients were removed to a pet-free environment or when the other pets were temporarily removed from the home.

One could argue correctly that this phenomenon does not necessarily demonstrate allergy, but rather some other mechanism, such as a neurotic behavior pattern toward another pet or person. Here again, however, until reliable, accurate information becomes available, one is fully justified in skin testing for dog and cat dander in nonseasonally allergic animals, if other animals also live in the same household.

My experience has been that pruritus resulting from neurotic behavior is unusual, although I vividly remember a boxer that was presented with a classic allergy history and clinical signs, that failed to respond to food trials and immunotherapy. In an attempt to determine whether allergens specific to the dog's own environment were involved, I hospitalized the dog for 3 days, during which time pruritus stopped and the skin gradually cleared. Convinced that the problem was caused by indigenous environmental allergens, I called the patient's owner to report my findings and asked that she take her dog home. When the client arrived, I spent about 5 minutes describing the dog's excellent progress and the steps to be taken next to find the offending allergen(s).

Before the owner arrived, the dog had been placed in a holding room next to the examining room, where he could easily hear our voices discussing the case. My assistant reported that, as soon as the dog heard his owner's voice, he began to scratch, and by the time he was brought out he was an excoriated mess. This was not only embarrassing to me, but upsetting to the client, until I was able to explain what had happened. The dog was then placed on a tranquilizer, which fortunately was effective in reducing the neurotic response.

In addition to cats and dogs, other pets in the house may possibly be responsible for reaction in the allergic pet. To date, no evidence proves that dogs have been allergic to rabbit, gerbil, or hamster fur, urine, or feces, but it is probably only a matter of time before the first case is reported. Because cedar shavings are the most common type of litter for pet rodents, one must also consider the possibility of allergy to this or other types of bedding.

In many species, such as the dog and horse, the dander shares common antigens with serum albumin. In the cat, the most important allergen, at least for man is the saliva deposited while grooming; the more the cat licks, the higher the probability of an allergic reaction in cat-sensitive individuals. Whether the dog reacts to the same antigens as man is unknown at this time and can only be assumed until definitive information becomes available.

Horsehair and Cattle Hair

The most difficult concept for most urban pet owners to understand is why animals who live in the city and have no direct contact with horses or cattle should be tested for these dangers. Although it is always good practice to explain the reason for specific procedures, compliance improves exponentially when the client understands the rationale for unfamiliar test and treatment procedures. Few people realize that carpets, old mattresses, oriental rugs, support webbing for older upholstered furniture, older types of felt carpet padding, and felt, as well as other materials, such as old wall plaster, may contain horsehair or cattle hairs. Horsehair is also used in the "backings" of suiting materials to give them additional body. Most men, in particular, when wearing a suit or sport jacket, have suddenly felt an annoying irritation at the back of their neck. If one feels for the source, one commonly pulls out a long black horsehair, which has been woven into the fabric to give it extra "body."

Additional allergens derived from animal danders that are occasionally involved in human allergy and could conceivably affect pets as well include *camel's hair, alpaca, angora, cashmere,* and *dried glues derived from the skin and tissues of horses and hogs.*

Obviously, this list is limited because the possibilities are endless. Until further studies are done, some of the foregoing will remain speculative and must await final clinical confirmation. In the meantime, all potential environmental allergens must be considered suspect, and every effort must be made to keep the patient's environment as free of allergens as possible.

SEASONAL PATTERNS

To summarize the interplay of environmental and aeroallergens, it is essential to think of the total environment as dynamic, with allergen loads rising and falling with the seasons and changing life styles. This interplay is best illustrated by Figure 8–2, typical of conditions in the mid-Atlantic states and areas with similar climatic conditions. One immediately sees that there are virtually no conditions under which only one allergen, or class of allergens, is present in the environment at any one time.

As shown in Figure 8–2, dust and indoor mold concentrations increase rapidly in early October, once heating systems and humidifiers are in use. These concentrations remain high throughout the winter and gradually diminish as spring approaches and furnaces are turned off, usually during April.

Outdoor molds begin to increase late in February or early in March, as the atmosphere warms and the frost and snow cover disappear. Mold concentrations then vary with climatic conditions, often reaching a peak in July, after which they begin to decline, only to peak again from late September to early December, as leaves drop and vegetation decays. Mold concentrations then drop precipitously following the first sustained frost and snow.

Trees begin to pollinate in early March; pollen concentrations peak rapidly and usually disappear by late May. Grasses usually start pollinating in early May and continue until late July, although grass pollen can actually be found throughout the summer and early fall, if climatic conditions are right and the temperature is warm enough.

English plantain also begins to pollinate by early May and continues at low levels, but in sufficient concentration to cause problems, throughout the summer and into November, unless there is a killing frost. Other weeds can pollinate throughout the summer, but the principal allergenic species begin early in August and continue through early October. By this time, the weather has usually turned cool enough to require heat occasionally, and the cycle continues.

Figure 8–2 quickly illustrates how complex the interrelationships among various allergens can become and how necessary it is to obtain a thorough medical history relative

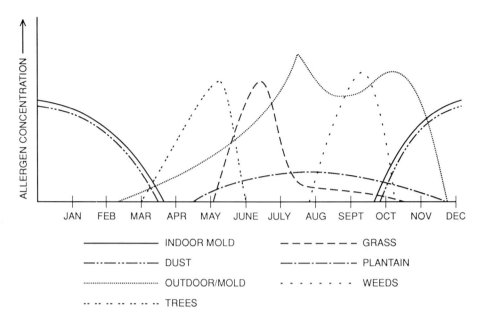

Fig. 8–2. Seasonal pattern of allergens in the mid-Atlantic states.

to seasonal variation in the intensity of clinical signs.

TREATMENT

In addition to standard skin testing and immunotherapy, discussed in Chapters 10 and 11, respectively, treatment consists of avoidance of the allergens wherever possible. Although it is impossible to eliminate dust, premises must be kept clean and dusted regularly. Vacuum cleaner bags should be checked regularly and changed frequently, to avoid dust buildup and leakage. Built-in vacuum systems, vented to the outside, provide the best protection against dust leakage from vacuum cleaners.

A good filtration system is also extremely important, and if the house has an existing hot-air heating system or central air conditioning, a central filtration system should be installed into the duct work. Otherwise, properly sized room filters can be used. One must remember, however, not only to install a good system, but to maintain and clean the filters regularly.

Ordinarily, dust-sensitive dogs respond well to treatment with commercial stock dust extracts obtained from the manufacturer. Occasionally, however, the patient does not improve and clinical signs persist or worsen during exposure to dust. In such cases, treatment with autogenous dust extract has been beneficial. It is increasingly difficult to find a source of autogenous dust, but some manufacturers of allergy extracts are still willing to prepare it. Otherwise, one must try to find a laboratory **licensed by the state,** with the knowledge and experience to prepare autogenous extracts. Dust should be collected according to the manufacturers' instructions and in collection bags supplied by them. In general, however, a fresh collection bag should be placed in the vacuum cleaner, and dust should be collected from various sources within the house, including rugs, draperies, baseboards, curtains, and mattresses. The principal disadvantages of autogenous dust are its high cost, and its limited effectiveness in some patients. If the patient's history and all clinical signs point to dust allergy, and if stock extracts do not seem to be working, however, an autogenous dust is often effective, and its use is justified under these conditions.

In summary, then, the general environment of every nonseasonal allergy patient must be thoroughly evaluated, if one expects to achieve maximum response to therapy.

REFERENCE
1. Scherago, M., Berkowitz, B., and Reitman, M.: Standardization of dust extracts. Ann. Allergy, *8*:437, 1950.

Preparation and Standardization
of Allergenic Extracts

All laboratories engaged in the interstate sale of allergenic extracts intended for use in man are licensed by the United States Food and Drug Administration (FDA). Extracts labeled for use in animals are manufactured and licensed under guidelines established by the Biologics Division of the United States Department of Agriculture. In actual practice, the products are identical, except for the label, and both are subject to rigorous inspection by these regulatory agencies. Identification, extraction, sterility testing, and standardization are the same for both products, to ensure that extracts meet the standards of both agencies. All aspects of the operation are reviewed regularly, from assurance that the proper pollens, mold spores, and other raw materials are used, through extraction, bottling, sterility, and labeling procedures. In essence, then, equivalent quality can be anticipated from any manufacturer holding both licenses.

PREPARATION OF ALLERGENS

Pollen is purchased from experienced collectors, skilled in the identification of allergenic plants, whereas mold spores may be cultured and harvested directly by the manufacturer or purchased from licensed mycology laboratories. Animal danders, feathers, and epidermals are purchased under contract and are collected from known, disease-free animals. In fact, the FDA now requires that all animals and birds from which source materials are obtained be placed under quarantine, and a veterinarian or his agent must certify the good health of these animals before the raw materials can be sold. Other allergens are obtained by a variety of recognized and approved procedures.

Following collection, the bulk allergens are inspected for quality and purity. All obvious foreign substances are removed, and the raw material is then defatted and dried.

The purpose of defatting is to prepare a water-soluble mass from which the allergenic principles can be removed by aqueous extraction. The extracts are then clarified by filtration and are concentrated by dialysis, after which their protein content is determined and final dilutions are prepared.

ANTIGENIC COMPONENTS

Pollen and molds do not contain a single antigen, but are complex mixtures, often with dozens of antigens (see Chap. 7). Not all are equally allergenic, however, and some are of little clinical significance. If the significant allergens of a specific pollen are known, they are usually eluted from the extract and constitute the bulk of the active principle of the final product. Because the significant allergens have not been identified for most spores and pollens, except for ragweed and a few others, the "crude" extract, containing all soluble antigens, is used for testing and treatment.

STANDARDIZATION UNITS

No single official unit of concentration is accepted by all allergists and government regulatory agencies. The two most widely used units of concentration for allergenic extracts are the weight/volume (w/v) and protein nitrogen units (PNU); both have their champions and detractors. The FDA has proposed a new standardization unit, the Allergy Unit, which has already been adopted for some antigens and will no doubt ultimately be adopted for all.

Ragweed is currently in a separate class and is standardized both in antigen E units, its most active allergenic component, and as either w/v or PNU.

To confuse matters more, the older literature refers to units of standardization no longer in use. The most confusing point of all, however, is that different units have virtually no relation to each other, so it is not possible to switch from one unit of standardization to another and expect to be using equipotent extracts.

Even extracts using the same standardization units vary in activity from batch to batch. This problem is not as marked in different batches using PNU standardization, but w/v extracts can vary widely. A 1:10 w/v batch of a particular pollen, for example, may contain 54,000 PNU, whereas another may have 137,000 PNU.

The following brief discussion of various standardization units is presented only so the veterinarian can become familiar with the different units used in both older and current literature.

NOON UNITS are referred to in the older literature and in some texts, but commercially available extracts are no longer labeled this way. This unit is a measure of the amount of allergen contained in one millionth of a grain of dry pollen, so one gram of pollen contains one million Noon units. As with all extracts, the activity varies from batch to batch because of variations in extraction methods and in concentration of allergens in different lots of pollen.

POLLEN UNITS are identical to Noon units.

TOTAL NITROGEN is a measure of the total milligrams of nitrogen in one milliliter of extract. Because this unit is a measure of all nitrogen and not just the nitrogen content of the allergenic protein, it does not necessarily reflect the true potency of the product.

PROTEIN NITROGEN UNITS are a measure of the nitrogen in the proteinaceous portion of the extract. This is probably more reproducible than some of the other standardization methods, and it is popular with many human and veterinary allergists. It also varies with extraction method, age of the extract, and protein content of the particular batch of pollen or other raw material, however. One PNU is equivalent to 0.00001 mg protein nitrogen. Converted into more common concentrations, 10,000 PNU are equivalent to 0.1 mg protein nitrogen.

WEIGHT BY VOLUME (w/v), the other standardization unit commonly used by many allergists, is a measure of the amount of defatted and dried allergen in a given volume of extract. A 1:100 concentration would be a 1% solution consisting of 1 gm protein per 100 ml. Here, too, variation in concentration among different batches of extracts can be great because of variables described for PNU. Consequently, the number of actual PNUs in each batch of w/v extracts can vary widely, increasing the potential for reactions when new batches are used.

One of the confusing aspects of working with w/v, as opposed to PNU, is the preparation of dilutions. A direct relation exists between the number of PNUs and the concentration. As PNU increases, the concentration becomes stronger. With w/v, on the other hand, it is just the reverse. The ratio is inverse, so as the ratio becomes higher, the concentration becomes more dilute. Therefore, a concentration of 20,000 PNU (0.2 mg) is twice as strong as one of 10,000 PNU (0.1 mg). A 1:100 w/v solution contains the antigen found in 1 gm allergenic substance, however, whereas a 1:1000 solution is 10 times more dilute and only contains the amount of antigen extracted from 0.1 gm. Therefore, until the clinician gains experience in using allergenic extracts, it is best to select one standardization method and use it as much as possible. I prefer to work with PNUs because dilutions are easier to calculate and the range of activity does not seem to be as wide from one batch to another.

PREPARATION OF DILUTIONS

Another area of confusion for some veterinarians is the preparation of dilutions of various extracts. A standard formula for dilution is:

$$V_1 C_1 = V_2 C_2$$

V_1 = the volume of concentrated extract
C_1 = the concentration of the stock extract
V_2 = the volume of the diluted extract
C_2 = the concentration of the diluted extract
In our example, we start with an extract containing a concentration of 63,000 PNU and want to make 3 ml of a 20,000-PNU dilution. V_1 is the only unknown. Therefore, substituting values,

$$V_1 = X \quad C_1 = 63,000$$
$$V_2 = 3 \quad C_2 = 20,000$$

therefore

$$63,000 \text{ X} = 3 \times 20,000, \text{ or } 60,000$$

60,000 divided by 63,0000 = 0.95 ml, to which must be added enough diluent (2.05 ml) to make 3 ml of a 20,000-PNU solution.

To simplify the process further, if the dilution to be made is divided by the higher concentration, the result will be the amount of concentrate needed to make one milliliter of dilution. This figure can then be multiplied by the number of milliliters to be made, and the proper amount of diluent can be added. For example, if you want to make 5 ml of a 20,000-PNU dilution from an 84,000-PNU concentrate, divide 20,000 by 84,000, giving you a value of 0.23 ml. Multiply by 5, which gives 1.19 ml (1.2 ml for practical purposes), to which is added a volume of diluent sufficient to make 5 ml.

SHELF LIFE

Most extracts are available as both aqueous and glycerinated solutions. Glycerinated extracts have the advantage of a much longer shelf life than the aqueous types, but they cannot be diluted and used for intradermal allergy skin testing because even dilute solutions may cause a false-positive reaction.

Other factors that can affect shelf life are dilution, temperature, and composition of the container. The more dilute the solution, the more likely it is to lose activity quickly. Removing extracts from the refrigerator and allowing them to sit at room temperature throughout the day also shortens the shelf life. Therefore, one should return the antigens to the refrigerator immediately after their use and take them out as needed. Finally, the bottles used, or recommended, by the manufacturer are treated to resist adsorption of the antigen onto the glass. If extracts are withdrawn and are then stored in untreated bottles, the probability of glass adsorption is greatly increased.

Another factor affecting potency is the concentration at which the extract is stored. The more dilute the solution, the more rapidly potency is lost through adsorption onto the glass container. It is also possible that the kinetics of biodegradation are increased as the solution becomes more dilute. Freezing must be avoided as it may cause precipitation of the protein allergen and a change in potency.

MODIFIED EXTRACTS

Over the years, attempts have been made to increase the safety and efficacy of allergenic extracts through the use of adjuvants, precipitation onto alum, emulsification of extracts, or transformation of their physical characteristics.

Adjuvants used in the past include incomplete Freund's adjuvant, peanut oil, and sodium alginate. None have withstood the test of time because of reactions or other treatment problems. In the 1960s, many practitioners will recall that an emulsified extract using mineral oil became available for veterinary use, with disastrous results. Innumerable cases of sterile abscesses, infected abscesses, and oil cysts occurred, causing grief for veterinarians, patients, and owners and the ultimate withdrawal of the product. This experience alone probably set veterinary allergy practice back at least 10 years, and some veterinarians still will not use immunotherapy because of problems encountered at that time.

The most successful modification, in my experience, has been the development of alum-adsorbed extracts. Two general types are available: (1) antigens prepared using normal extraction processes and then adsorbed onto alum; and (2) a pyridine-extracted, alum-precipitated antigen, marketed under the trade name Allpyral by Hollister-Stier (West Haven, CT). Alum-precipitated extracts slow absorption in much the same way as emulsions, resulting in a slower, more sustained antigen stimulation. My own experience in investigating the use of Allpyral for several years was extremely favorable, with an excellent overall response using a nine-injection series.

Much research is in progress on the next generation of allergenic extracts. The goal of current research is to make the extracts purer by identifying the antigens actually involved in an allergic reaction, and by eliminating extraneous antigens. Another major research effort under way is attempting to find ways to modify the molecular structure of antigens to increase potency and efficacy while reducing adverse reactions. Among the compounds under investigation are allergoids, urea-denatured antigens, and polymerized antigens that have been modified by binding to chemical agents, such as formalin, urea, glutaraldehyde, polyethylene glycol, and similar compounds.

10 ‖ *Allergy Skin Testing*

Technically, allergy skin testing is a simple procedure—the interpretation of the test can sometimes be difficult. Yet anyone who has ever performed tuberculin tests, or given an intradermal injection, can do allergy skin tests. All it takes is a little practice, a lot of self-confidence, and acceptance of the inevitability of mistakes in the beginning and, occasionally, throughout your allergy practice career. The most important things to know are

(1) which allergic patients to test;
(2) what to expect from testing and immunotherapy;
(3) which antigens to use in your particular practice area;
(4) which standardization concentration to use; and
(5) how to conduct a proper test.

SELECTION OF PATIENTS

Not every allergic pet is a candidate for allergy skin testing and immunotherapy, and a treatment program is doomed to failure unless certain factors are taken into consideration.

First is a thorough understanding by the client of what is being done and what you are trying to accomplish. It is vitally important that expectations not exceed reality; the client must fully understand that even with a perfect allergy history and clear, well-defined skin test reactions, not every patient responds to immunotherapy.

Of course, the veterinarian must also be convinced that skin testing and injection therapy are the proper approach to the management of inhalant allergy. A veterinarian who vacillates and does not appear certain when recommending testing and injection therapy convinces neither the client nor himself of the wisdom of his approach.

A second consideration is compliance of the client. Most veterinarians develop good instincts about their clients and know which will cooperate and follow a program and which will not. Unless the client will follow all management instructions and will return regularly for immunotherapy and re-evaluation, one should treat the patient medically and forget a biologic approach.

A third consideration is patient's age, which in itself is not a contraindication to testing. There is little point, however, in testing and treating an aged dog, arbitrarily 13 or older, because by the time the tests are performed and immunotherapy is completed, the dog will have come close to its anticipated life expectancy and will have little time to enjoy the benefits of treatment. In the cat, the age is higher because of their greater longevity. Of course, these statements are generalities, and the decision to test and treat must ultimately be made on an individual basis.

FACTORS AFFECTING RESPONSE TO TESTING AND IMMUNOTHERAPY

Ordinarily, one can reasonably anticipate a 75 to 78% good-to-excellent response, if the skin tests are carefully performed and immunotherapy is properly administered. This response rate still leaves about 20% that either show no improvement whatsoever or only partially improve. Here again, a number of factors may be involved.

The first is improper preparation of the patient, discussed in more detail later in this chapter. Essentially, the problem arises when insufficient time elapses between the last dose of corticosteroids, antihistamines, or tranquilizers and the administration of the allergy skin test. The selection of improper sedatives for fractious or nervous animals can also affect the reliability of the test procedure.

Other factors include the time interval between testing and reading, the potency of the test and treatment extracts, the definitiveness of the test reaction sites, and the person who administers the immunotherapy. A significant cause of treatment failure is the lack of recognition of other important causes of pruritic skin disease, such as food allergy or parasites. An immunotherapy program cannot succeed if the patient has not been evaluated thoroughly for all possible causes of the problem.

As expected, the fuzzier the reaction and the more judgmental one must be in classifying it, the higher the probability of a poor response to treatment.

Finally, a few patients inexplicably fail to respond to skin tests, regardless of testing techniques, allergic status, or pretesting preparation. Whether this failure is due to anergy or to a combination of factors is uncertain. These patients present special problems in that they may require retesting several times at monthly intervals before positive reactions are seen. One may also need to test these patients at different times of the year, or even to make a presumptive diagnosis and begin immunotherapy, selecting the most probable antigens based on the patient's history. In such a patient, one could justifiably try in vitro testing.

WHEN TO TEST

No consensus exists on whether to test during the allergy season (co-seasonally) or afterwards (extraseasonally). If the allergy is nonseasonal, of course, one has no choice. For the seasonally sensitive patient, however, the decision must be based on personal experience and the recommendation of veterinary allergists.

I have had seasonally allergic patients that tested poorly during the allergy season, but had good reactions a month or more after the season was over. I have also had others that tested poorly out of season, but had good reactions when tested during the allergy season. Still others had equally good or bad reactions regardless of when testing was done. Ultimately, the decision must be based on the patient's circumstances. In general, it is best to test when patients are available, in other words, when they are having trouble. Unfortunately, with many clients, out of

sight means definitely out of mind, and as soon as the worst of the allergy problem is over, it is forgotten until the following year.

ANTIGEN SELECTION

To the emerging veterinary allergist, nothing can be more confusing than selecting the proper antigens for skin testing and treatment. Faced with a bewildering array of potential allergens, it is no wonder that many veterinarians recoil in dismay and revert to steroids or some other form of therapy.

Fortunately, the challenge is not as formidable as it initially seems. One's first decision is how complete or extensive to make the antigen test list. A screening procedure, testing only for *major allergens*, identifies some patients, but leaves many undiagnosed. If the *significant allergens* are then added to the list, a much larger number of allergies will be identified. Adding the *minor allergens* identifies a few more patients, but is probably not cost effective, except for the veterinary allergist or veterinarians establishing themselves as local or regional reference centers. Major, significant, and minor allergens vary from region to region, and antigen selections can be based on the significance in allergy found in the tables in Chapter 7. Allergens assigned a number 4 rating are considered major, numbers 3 and 2 are significant, whereas number 1 is of minor importance. Mold selection can be based on the tables in Chapter 7 or from the group listed in the suggested universal starter set in Table 10–1.

Determining which allergens to include in an initial test program is the most difficult decision. Future additions and deletions are much easier and are based on observation and experience with patients. To approach the problem rationally, it probably makes most sense for the novice allergist to select about 25 to 30 antigens as a base and, as experience is gained and the allergy practice dictates, to proceed by gradually adding more test antigens. Selection of additional antigens can be made on the same basis as that used for selecting the initial group, as well as on recommendations from technical representatives of the various manufacturers of allergy extracts and from local physician allergists.

Table 10–1. Suggested Antigens for Inclusion in a Universal Starting Test Set

Environmental Agents	Trees	Grasses	Weeds
Dust	Elm	Timothy	Cocklebur
Dust mite	Black walnut	Fescue	Indigenous ragweed
Kapok	Local oak	June	Lamb's-quarters
Wool	Sycamore	Rye	Pigweed
Feathers	Mulberry		English plantain

Molds

Botrytis	Phoma
Curvularia	Aureobasidium (Pullularia)
Epicoccum	Rhizopus
Helminthosporium	Rhodotorula
Cladosporium (Hormodendrum)	Stemphylium
Mucor	

My recommendations for a universal starting test list are given in Table 10–1. Allergens found only in low density in the veterinarian's specific practice area can be eliminated, whereas locally important allergens should be included. For example, Bermuda grass is an important allergen in most areas of the country, but not in those northern states in which it is too cold for them to survive. In the West, the pollens of olive and hazelnut trees are also important sensitizers and should be included in any basic set of test extracts for that area.

A test program is dynamic and subject to change and should not be considered static and "etched in stone." Over the years, my list of test antigens has changed many times, and it is still changing. As pollen and mold spore counts are followed, those seen frequently or in locally high concentration are added to the test list. On the other hand, it may not be cost effective to continue to test with allergens to which few animals react, so these may be replaced in the test program by more productive antigens.

Flexibility, then, becomes the key. The test and treatment program should be reviewed periodically by evaluating the number of positive skin-test reactions obtained and patients' response to therapy. Changes can then be made rationally, based on your own clinical experience.

TEST MIXTURES

Test extracts are available both as individual antigens and as mixtures. Unless strong cross-reactivity among antigens in the mixture is known to exist—and even here it is still better not to use them, mixtures should not be used in order to prevent the following potential problems:

1. The higher the number of antigens in a mixture, the lower the concentration of each test antigen. For example, if a 1000-protein nitrogen unit (PNU) test solution contains 10 antigens, such as tree antigens, only 100 PNU of each antigen will actually be present in the mixture. This number may be below the patient's threshold level of response to the antigens, and positive reactions may be missed.

2. Little cross-reactivity exists among the various species of trees, molds, and most weeds, so the inadequate amount of antigen, without the reinforcement of cross-reactivity, reduces the reliability of the test even further. Therefore, one should avoid using the 10-tree mix, the weed mixes, and the 4-mold mixes commonly available.

3. Among the inhalants, grasses are the most cross-antigenic of the botanic groups. Consequently, a 7-grass mix is another commonly available test antigen. Of all mixtures, this is most likely to give reliable test reactions and the only one for which an argument can be made for its use. In spite of the group's cross-antigenicity, however, negative reactions often occur in grass-sensitive patients. Yet the same patients frequently elicit positive reactions when tested with individual grasses from the group.

3. Another problem with test mixtures is that we have no way of knowing which specific allergen is responsible for a positive re-

action, unless individual tests are also run. This problem, in turn, raises the important question, "without specific allergen identification, which antigen(s) will be used for immunotherapy?" When treatment is instituted with an allergen mixture, instead of individual allergens, one always risks introducing extraneous antigens for which there is no need. Even more important, the amount of allergen in each treatment injection is diluted according to the number found in the mix, thereby reducing the amount of available antigen in each treatment and increasing the time needed to reach the optimum therapeutic dose.

DOSE AND STRENGTH OF TEST ANTIGENS

Only aqueous antigens, *without glycerin,* should be used for intradermal skin testing because even minute amounts of glycerin can cause false-positive reactions. The two most common strengths for intradermal tests are 1000 PNU/ml and a 1:1000 w/v dilution. Because we cannot actually compare the relative potency of the two standardization units, it is best to adopt one or the other, to gain experience in the type of reactions to be expected during skin testing and treatment. Although the actual potency varies from batch to batch with either extract, PNU standardization is more likely to be consistent than w/v.

Test extracts may either be purchased commercially in 5-ml vials, or the veterinarian may prepare them fresh from stock concentrates. Until the allergy practice is large enough to justify the substantial investment in stock concentrates, it is more realistic to purchase test antigens initially. The number of tests can be modified, discarded, or added to with minimal outlay. Once the allergy practice has been established, stock concentrates can be purchased and test dilutions made as needed.

I test with 1000-PNU concentrations and have found these satisfactory for evaluating my patients. On occasion, I find it necessary to test with more dilute solutions, particularly if an inordinate number of patients show positive reactions to a particular antigen, but standard concentrations of stock antigens usually effectively elicit positive reactions.

The most common procedure for intradermal skin testing is to inject 0.05 ml of the test concentration into the superficial epidermal layers of the patient's skin. In my skin tests, I use an even smaller dose and inject between 0.02 and 0.03 ml intradermally. By using a lower volume of the test antigen, I feel more certain not only that these positive reactions are true positive reactions, but also that they represent important allergens for the patient. Occasional references in the veterinary literature, and particularly older reports, recommend injecting 0.1 ml of 1500- or 2000-PNU concentration for routine intradermal skin testing. No justification exists for using this volume or concentration because the number of false-positive reactions is increased markedly both by irritation and by sheer fluid volume.

CONDUCTING THE TEST

Allergy skin testing requires a measure of skill that must be developed, but the techniques of intradermal injection and test-site evaluation can be learned by any veterinarian. What is required is intellectual curiosity and the patience to spend time performing multiple test injections and readings. Most veterinarians have at least had some experience performing tuberculin tests or administering intradermal vaccines. If not, one should practice on a cadaver until experience is gained in administering consistently uniform injections. Competence in reading and interpreting the tests only comes after enough tests have been evaluated and compared with both the patient's history and response to therapy.

Before beginning an allergy testing program, a number of procedural recommendations and general precautions should be followed, to ensure the best possible results.

Preparation of Patients

Proper preparation of the patient is of prime importance in performing allergy skin tests, and failure to attend to even small details can adversely affect the result. The following recommendations are presented in no particular order; all are equally important.

Discontinuance of Corticosteroids and Other Drugs

If the patient has been receiving glucocorticoids, these drugs must be withdrawn before one administers the tests. Because the duration of effect varies so widely among the different corticosteroids, ranging from hours for prednisolone to days for betamethasone, firm recommendations cannot be made for the time interval to elapse between the last dose of steroid and the beginning of the tests. Recommendations vary among veterinary allergists, but a good rule of thumb is to wait 2 weeks for each month the patient has received the steroid, depending on the type used. If the patient has been treated with repository or other long-acting corticosteroids, an even longer interval may be required. I have seen at least one dog whose skin-test reactions were nondiagnostic until steroids had been discontinued for about 6 months.

Steroids apparently have no effect on skin-test results in man. Therefore, when reading the human literature, one must remember that the information relating to steroids cannot be extrapolated directly to the dog. Information on the inhibitory effect of these drugs in the cat, horse, and cow is insufficient.

All antihistamines and phenothiazine-based tranquilizers should be discontinued for at least 3 days, and preferably a week, before skin testing. In fact, a recent study showed that some antihistamines could obliterate, or at least diminish, skin-test reactions for up to 9 days.

Sedation and Anesthesia

Sedatives or anesthetics are rarely necessary in skin testing. If they are used, however, one must avoid narcotics, barbiturates, or the phenothiazine-based tranquilizers. Many years ago, before we were fully aware of the effects of barbiturates on skin tests, a colleague and I completely wiped out the reactions in a dog used to demonstrate skin-testing techniques and positive skin tests. The effect was so profound that the dog would not even react to the highest concentration of histamine available for use as a positive control.

To date, the only tranquilizer studied and shown not to interfere with skin-test reactions is xylazine (Rompum), and the only indication for such use is in fractious, nervous, or "jumpy" dogs.

AVOID STRUGGLING WITH, EXCITING, OR FIGHTING WITH THE PATIENT AS MUCH AS POSSIBLE because this releases epinephrine, which may be at a high enough level to interfere with skin tests. If the patient cannot be kept calm, one should use xylazine to keep him relaxed. If struggling does occur, and if the skin-test reactions are poor, the test should be repeated on another day, using xylazine. If, on the other hand, good positive reactions are obtained, retesting should not be necessary.

A report on a study presented at the 1989 meeting of the Academy of Veterinary Dermatology confirmed that xylazine did not interfere with allergy skin tests. The results of the study also showed that acepromazine did not block the development of positive skin-test reactions when the drug was used as a sedative. Even though test sites were not obliterated, however, all reactions were reduced in size, when compared with those of control subjects. Therefore, because many dogs already have reduced or weak skin-test reactions as a result of prior medications or unknown factors, reducing the reaction further could result in the classification of positive reactions as negative. Consequently, xylazine is the compound of choice when a sedative is required to calm a nervous or difficult patient.

Testing Sites

The lateral lumbar area and chest wall are the most suitable sites for allergy skin testing. Not only are these areas easily accessible during the actual administration of the test, but results can also be read on the floor, if necessary, especially in nervous or fractious patients. Moreover, dogs in sternal or lateral recumbency usually relax more quickly and require less restraint than dogs forced to lie on their backs.

Occasionally, reports in the literature recommended testing on the animal's inner thighs or abdomen, but these sites have little to recommend them. For one thing, the dog must be rolled over for adequate exposure, and even calm dogs often fight and resist being turned on their backs with their legs extended. Consequently, dogs needing minimal restraint under ordinary circumstances may require many restraining sets of hands to complete the skin tests. Reading the test sites, of course, presents the same problems. Finally, we do not know whether these are really good sites for conducting a skin test. In man, for example, the back and upper arm seem to be more reliable for testing than the abdomen. The same may or may not be true for animal patients. What we do know is that the lateral lumbar area and chest wall have been reliably used for many years, and until studies determine the location of better sites, we see no reason to change.

Select a site as free of lesions as possible. Nodules, papules, crusts, scales, inflammation, and excoriations not only complicate reading of skin-test sites, but also they can suppress the response or entirely eliminate it. In a severe case with extensive lesions, finding one patch of skin large enough to conduct the tests may be difficult. In such cases, it may be necessary to test at multiple sites, wherever patches of relatively unaffected skin can be found. In rare cases, it may even be necessary to institute a *VERY* short course of steroids and antihistamines, to clear up enough skin to run the tests.

If multiple test sites are used, each site should be accompanied by a negative control injection. Multiple negative control injections should also be used if a large number of tests are administered. In such cases, individual species (trees, weeds) should be grouped together and a negative control used for each group.

Skin Preparation

The patient's hair should be gently clipped as close to the skin as possible, without traumatizing it. Depilatories may be used a few days before the actual skin test is scheduled; the disadvantage is that the patient must be handled twice, and if irritation occurs, the test will have to be postponed.

There is usually no need to wash the skin, unless it is particularly greasy or dirty. If the skin must be washed, wash it gently with a *VERY* bland or mild soap. Work up a lather,

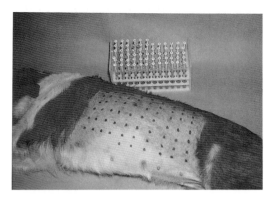

Fig. 10–1. Marking of skin-test sites. (Courtesy of Dr. John M. MacDonald, Auburn University School of Veterinary Medicine, Auburn, Alabama.)

rinse with warm water, and pat it dry. Alcohol or other germicides are not necessary, and at least one reference source suggests that alcohol may actually interfere with skin-test reactions.

Once the skin has been prepared, test sites are marked with a felt or laundry pen (Fig. 10–1). The marking procedure is optional and can consist of a row of dots with the injection made above, below, or to the right of it, or it can be a group of squares with the injections placed in the center. The only purpose of marking the sites is to identify which test is which, so it can be accurately recorded.

Finally, handle the skin gently when testing; be careful not to pinch or irritate the skin unnecessarily. The skin test is based on the injected antigen binding to its antigen-specific immunoglobulin E (IgE) antibody attached to a skin mast cell. This process then sets off the reaction leading to degranulation and the release of histamine and other mediators, resulting in the wheal and inflammation indicative of a positive skin test. Rough handling may traumatize the mast cells and may cause them to degranulate, so not only may they be incapable of reacting, but also the inflammation caused by the released mediators may create a false-positive reaction.

Skin Testing

Intradermal Testing

The intradermal (intracutaneous) skin test is the test of choice in animals, both for re-

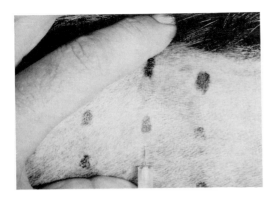

Fig. 10–2.   Proper angle of syringe for allergy skin testing. (Courtesy of Dr. John M. MacDonald, Auburn University School of Veterinary Medicine, Auburn, Alabama.)

liability and reproducibility. Using a 1-ml syringe calibrated in increments of 0.01 ml, hold it almost parallel to the skin, with the bevel of the needle up, so any antigen excess will be directed superficially, rather than deep (Figs. 10–2 and 10–3). Be sure the syringe is free of air because injected air interferes with an accurate reading. Then inject 0.02 to 0.03 ml (virtually a drop) of the antigen into the most superficial layers of the epidermis. Injected air is easily recognized; it seems to "spread" in the skin and gives the skin a blanched appearance.

If tuberculin syringes are used, a $\frac{3}{8}$- to $\frac{5}{8}$-inch needle with a 27-gauge bore should be selected; however, special 1-ml "allergist's" syringes, with a flat-ended, rather than tapered, barrel and a needle fused onto the syringe, reduce dead space in the barrel, minimize air-bubble formation, and improve control over the size of the injection (Fig.

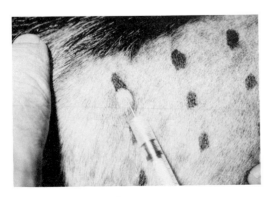

Fig. 10–3.   Characteristic bleb raised during skin testing. (Courtesy of Dr. John M. MacDonald, Auburn University School of Veterinary Medicine, Auburn, Alabama.)

10–4). Syringes are available in "allergist tray packs" of 25, from both B-D and Terumo.

Because of its sensitivity and the increased possibility of severe reactions in man, intradermal testing is usually reserved for special circumstances in human medicine. A number of other skin tests used in man that are not effective in animals are described here briefly, so they will be recognizable when one reads the human literature.

Prick Puncture and Pressure Testing

The most popular skin test in human medicine today is the prick puncture test because it is safer and less likely to provoke systemic reactions than intradermal testing. It is also sensitive, correlates closely with the patient's history and clinical signs, and is less tedious to perform. In this procedure, a drop of antigen is placed on the skin, and one passes a sterile needle through the drop. The skin is barely punctured, then is picked up, as in a smallpox vaccination.

The prick pressure test is a variant in which a drop of antigen is placed on the skin; a needle then depresses the skin through the drop of antigen and then picks at the skin as it comes out.

Scratch Testing

Another test used in human medicine in the past, and one that had a vogue in veterinary medicine as well, is the scratch test. A drop of antigen is placed on the skin, and a scarifier is drawn through the drop, barely scratching the skin without drawing blood (Fig. 10–5).

In addition to the foregoing, a number of scarifying devices have been developed over the years, in an attempt to automate testing, to provide for consistent, uniform depth of skin penetration, or to reduce discomfort. None have achieved widespread use, and all have been abandoned by most clinicians.

Over the years, I have tried many of these devices in dogs, with inconsistent results. If proper test antigens could be developed for animal use, such devices would have great potential in veterinary medicine because they would produce uniform, consistent tests with minimal discomfort and maximum reproducibility.

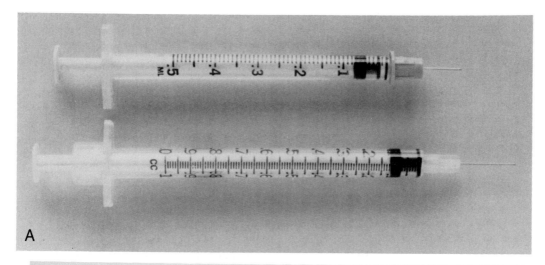

A

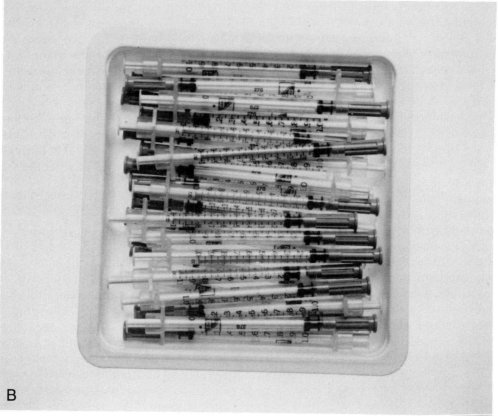

B

Fig. 10–4. A. "Allergist's" syringe, 0.5 and 1.0 ml. B. Packaging tray. (Courtesy of Becton Dickinson.)

This brings us back full circle to the intradermal test, the most diagnostically reliable skin test for use in animals. To ensure maximum diagnostic value from the test, certain precautions and procedures must be followed.

Always use fresh solutions. If you purchase your test antigens and suspect that you are not seeing enough positive, or as many strongly positive, reactions in suspect cases, obtain fresh solutions. Under any circumstances, you should probably replace the antigens 2 to 3 months before their expiration date. If you prepare your own solutions, use

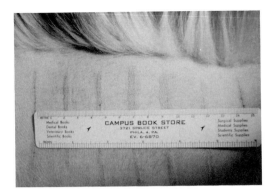

Fig. 10–5. Scratch test in a dog.

concentrates with current dating, and prepare fresh extracts every few months.

Always use a positive and a negative control, for reference points for comparison of test injections. Actually, you should use two positive controls: a 1:10,000 concentration of histamine phosphate solution for intradermal skin testing and a known mast-cell histamine releaser. The best histamine releaser is compound 48/80. Unfortunately, this compound is a research chemical and is not available for routine use. Therefore, one must use a good substitute, such as a dilute morphine solution, which can be prepared easily from morphine injection or morphine hypodermic tablets (HTs).

An HT dissolved in 1 ml saline, or the stock morphine injection solution, is the base from which dilutions are made, and histamine is the control to which it is compared. Inject a drop of the histamine control intradermally, and measure the maximum diameter reached. Then prepare serial 10-fold dilutions of the morphine solution, using the same phenolsaline diluent used in the allergenic extracts and supplied by the manufacturer. Inject a drop of each of the dilutions intradermally, adjacent to the histamine control, until the wheal size is equivalent to that of the histamine control.

The reason for using morphine, or any histamine releaser, is that it can initiate mast-cell degranulation, demonstrating the functional capability of the cell. If only histamine is used, it may indicate the potential size of the wheal, but it tells nothing of the capability of mast cells to release histamine. Inhibition of mast-cell degranulation can result

from pharmacologic inhibitors, mast-cell exhaustion, anergy, or other factors. When a negative or minimal reaction is obtained with the morphine control, or any other histamine releaser, there is no purpose in conducting the test that day because negative responses will be meaningless. Retest on a monthly basis until a positive reaction occurs. This process may take weeks to months in a pharmacologically suppressed patient.

The negative control should be the same as the fluid used for diluting the test extracts and should be obtained from the same manufacturer from which the antigens or bulk extracts are purchased.

Injection sites must be uniform. If a poor injection is made, cross out that site, move to the next one, and repeat the test injection before continuing.

Start reading the tests about 5 minutes after giving the injection; some dogs exhibit reactions quickly, whereas others may be slow. Although the average dog develops maximum reactions in about 15 minutes, at which point reactions slowly start to fade, I have had many dogs in which even the positive controls developed early and had started to fade by the end of 15 minutes. If, as some literature suggests, you wait 15 to 30 minutes before beginning to read test sites, many positive reactions will be missed.

On occasion, especially with mold allergy, reactions may not develop for several hours, or even 24 hours, after the injection. Initial reactions may also fade, only to reappear later. These late-phase reactions are difficult to explain and may be due to a subclass of IgG, rather than IgE. No evidence at this time suggests that they represent an increased state of hypersensitivity; rather, they are probably a reaction variant. Reactions developing 24 hours later, or more, may even represent delayed, tuberculin-type reactions. Many molds and bacteria, for example, have induced both type I (IgE-mediated) and type IV (cell-mediated) responses.[1]

Bacterial tests are read differently and are covered in Chapter 16.

Positive skin-test reactions do not resemble those seen in man, except perhaps for those seen in infants. In man, one sees wheals with irregular projections, surrounded by a

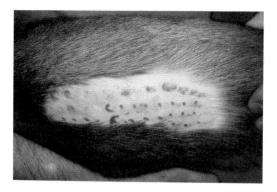

Fig. 10–6. Positive skin-test reaction in the dog.

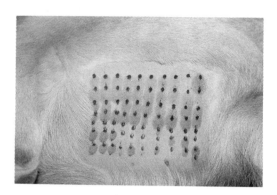

Fig. 10–8. Positive skin-test reaction in the dog. (Courtesy of Dr. John M. MacDonald, Auburn University School of Veterinary Medicine, Auburn, Alabama.)

zone of erythema, the so-called wheal-and-flare reaction with pseudopods. In the dog, reactions are discrete, steep-walled, and reddened (Figs. 10–6 to 10–8), except in dogs under 8 months old, whose reactions are generally small and hard to read. Reaction sites in children are also smaller and more poorly defined than in adults.

Positive reactions are also poorly defined in the cat. In fact, reactions in the cat may be so small and difficult to read that they often require an interpretative evaluation and frequent use of "judgment calls."

The test injection site should be compared with both the negative and positive controls, and it should be at least 2 mm larger than the negative control to be considered positive. Grading reactions is not necessary, except as an indication of relative sensitivity. In general, the larger the reaction, the greater the degree of sensitivity. This rule is far from absolute, however. Because many factors can

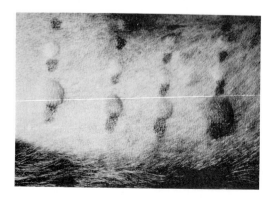

Fig. 10–7. Positive skin-test reaction in the dog. (Courtesy of Dr. John M. MacDonald, Auburn University School of Veterinary Medicine, Auburn, Alabama.)

affect the reaction size, a patient may have small reactions, yet clinically be highly sensitive.

Test sites are usually distinguishable and present few reading problems. Some dogs are not strong reactors, however, whereas others occasionally produce reactions that are not easy to interpret. When visual interpretation is uncertain, judgment can be improved by palpation and the use of side light. Gently compare the positive and negative test sites with the tips of the fingers of one hand, while you feel the questionable test sites with the finger tip of the other hand. Positive tests should be turgid and should feel larger than the negative control site. Gentle palpation is stressed; too much pressure or manipulation may cause degranulation of mast cells and false positive results. Side light may also help to confirm positive reactions. With the lights dim, hold a small flashlight parallel to the skin, with the light shining across the test sites. Observe whether shadows are cast; then compare them to the control sites, the definitively positive reactions, and those judged to be positive by palpation.

The use of certain blue dyes can also be of value to the novice allergist. Although Evans blue is the best known dye for the use in allergy, trypan blue, which had a considerable vogue in the 1960s as a treatment for demodectic mange, also works well and is suitable if it can be found. Just prior to skin testing, depending on the size of the patient, 1 or 2 ml of the dyes are injected intravenously, which then becomes bound to serum

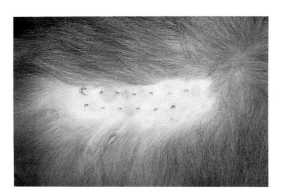

Fig. 10–9.   Positive skin-test reaction in the dog as evidenced by blue dye.

albumin. When a positive reaction occurs, mediators are released, causing capillary dilatation and increased capillary permeability. The protein-bound dye is extravasated with the edema fluid at the site of a positive reaction, presenting a dramatic blue indicator of the reaction (Fig. 10–9).

From the foregoing, it is obvious that allergy skin testing is not a difficult procedure, but one that requires attention to details. Before embarking on an allergy program, however, one must remember that, even though test solutions are moderately priced, they can be expensive if unused. Therefore, unless a veterinarian is prepared to become proficient and to perform enough tests to justify the investment in materials, it would be better to refer the case to someone who tests patients for allergy on a regular basis.

IN VITRO TESTS

At this writing, a recommendation cannot be made for or against in vitro tests. Comparative evaluations based on skin tests alone are difficult to make because in vitro tests measure serum antibody, whereas skin tests measure mast-cell bound antibody. Both radioallergosorbent tests (RAST) and enzyme-linked immunosorbent assay (ELISA) could be of great value to the clinician, if these methods prove to be diagnostically reliable, especially in nervous or fractious dogs or in those whose skin is so damaged that reliable test results cannot be expected. My principal objections at this point are the use of test mixtures, the cost, the limited flexibility in testing (you must use the manufacturer's test antigens), and the unavailability of results for several days, whereas with skin testing, results are known immediately.

REFERENCE

1. Rajka, G.: Studies in hypersensitivity to molds and staphylococci in prurigo Besnier (atopic dermatitis). Acta Derm. Venereol. (Stockholm), *43 (Suppl. 54)*:43, 1963.

Immunotherapy

Immunotherapy (hyposensitization, desensitization, allergy injections) is used in an attempt to induce a state of tolerance in patients, so they can then be exposed to the offending allergen(s) with minimal or no discomfort. **IMMUNOTHERAPY IS NOT A SUBSTITUTE FOR AVOIDANCE,** which is still the best means of obtaining relief from allergy. Avoidance is not always possible in the dog or cat, however, because it is virtually impossible totally to control their movement. Moveover, no practical way exists to prevent them from sniffing the ground, plants, and flowers.

THEORETIC CONSIDERATIONS

Tolerance is induced by giving injections of increasing higher doses of allergenic extracts, so the patient gradually develops resistance to the offending allergen(s). The actual process is not clearly understood. Not too many years ago we would have said unequivocally that improvement was due to the development of blocking antibody, an antibody of the immunoglobulin G (IgG) class that, theoretically, combines with the allergen and blocks or prevents it from binding with mast cell or basophil-bound IgE.

Several problems are associated with the blocking-antibody theory. Although blocking antibody probably plays some role in the management of allergic disease, it is becoming increasingly obvious that the immunotherapy story is more complex. For example, not all dogs or people undergoing successful immunotherapy have an increase in IgG levels. Furthermore, the blocking-antibody theory does not explain certain clinical observations, such as the marked improvement occasionally seen following allergy skin testing or shortly after the first dose of an immunotherapy series. As discussed later in this chapter, my treatment procedure consists of dividing all the positive reactors into

small groups and giving a series of gradually increasing doses of each group. Within 24 to 48 hours of receiving the **first** dose of the injection series, a dose that represents only about 25 to 30% of the positive skin-test reactions, the patient becomes asymptomatic and remains so for a week or longer. Obviously, time has not been sufficient for blocking antibody to develop, certainly not to the allergens that have not yet been given, so the effect must be due to something else. We now know that other factors are also apparently involved in the response to immunotherapy, such as a decrease in antigen-specific IgE antibodies, an apparent decrease in the mast-cell response to antibody stimulation, and the generation of allergen-specific suppressor T cells. Moreover, in time, additional factors may also be found, as our understanding of this complex process becomes clearer.

One can logically ask, "why will allergens entering the body via natural routes cause allergy, while the same antigens given parenterally help to prevent it?" The truth is that we really do not know. Theoretically, in the genetically programmed allergic individual, inhaled allergens crossing mucosal and other natural barriers, do so in **RELATIVELY** small numbers. These allergens are then "processed" by submucosal macrophages and are presented to the proper lymphocytes for antigen production, with IgE the most common antibody produced. During immunotherapy, on the other hand, antigens are given in much higher concentration by an unnatural route, such as a parenteral injection. These antigens are apparently processed "differently," producing IgG-blocking antibody while concurrently altering the other immune responses discussed previously.

WHY MORE VETERINARIANS DO NOT USE IMMUNOTHERAPY

In spite of the well-documented benefits of allergy immunotherapy, many veterinarians are still reluctant to initiate a test-and-treatment program. The reasons for this reluctance are complex and multifactored and include the following:

1. Many veterinarians have been stung by exaggerated claims for test-and-treatment "kits" in the past, only to find that their expectations exceeded reality. Consequently, "once burned is twice warned," and they have been reluctant to become involved again.

2. Some veterinarians are uncertain how to initiate and develop an immunotherapy program. Fear can be the most enervating influence in life, and the only way to overcome it is to begin testing and treating patients. By following the procedures and recommendations in the earlier chapters of this book, any veterinarian should be able to begin an allergy therapy program.

3. A third reason that many veterinarians are reluctant to institute a program is the low response rates frequently reported for allergy testing and immunotherapy, often as low as 40%. One would certainly have to agree that if a 40 to 50% good-to-excellent response rate was the best that could be expected, it would hardly justify the time and expense spent in working up and treating the patient. Many of these reports have come from veterinarians with insufficient experience in clinical allergy, from veterinarians using an insufficient number of test antigens, and from institutions and clinics that do not administer their own immunotherapy. These clinics regularly dispense treatment vials to clients and rely on them to store the extracts properly, to administer the injections, and to report back accurately. In many cases, no direct post-treatment clinical evaluation of the patient is made, and surveys of clients are used as the basis for efficacy. In fact, independent retrospective reviews of patients by me, as well as by other veterinary allergists, have shown that a 75 to 78% good-to-excellent response rate is a reasonable expectation. In our studies, this meant no more than a rare uncomfortable day, without maintenance corticosteroids or antihistamines for support.

4. Finally, many veterinarians have convinced themselves that clients are not interested in good medicine and are only looking for a steroid type of "quick fix" or "magic bullet." This view is delusionary, at best, because most clients are sophisticated and are aware of the other treatment options available to them. They read the medical reports in newspapers and magazines, are aware of the side effects of corticosteroids and other drugs, and know that allergy skin testing and "shots" are a more than viable alternative. Given the option, many clients opt for specific immunotherapy and refuse corticosteroids, even though they know that not every pet responds.

INITIATING THERAPY

A positive skin-test reaction merely indicates the presence of a skin-sensitizing IgE antibody, but it gives no information on whether an actual clinical sensitivity exists. Consequently, we have no unequivocal recommendation for choosing particular positive skin-test antigens for the treatment program. In human medicine, most allergists recommend treating only with those allergens for which the patient's medical history indicates clear-cut evidence of sensitivity. Unfortunately, this recommendation is much more realistic for man than for animals, as we are rarely able to obtain the degree of historical confirmation necessary to make such a rational decision in our animal patients.

Because many allergens are concurrent (see Tables 7–1 to 7–3 and Fig. 8–2), the only way to identify clinical sensitivity positively is to conduct a provocative challenge test. This is easier said than done because the patient must be placed in an aerosol chamber, which is then insufflated with an aerosolized allergen, after which the patient is watched to see whether a reaction occurs. This procedure is obviously impractical. It would be necessary to challenge the patient with each of the skin-test-positive allergens and to stop the test as soon as a reaction occurred. Because only one positive reaction could be permitted in any one day, and because several days would have to elapse between challenge sessions, the provocative challenge could take weeks or months. In a more practical vein, experience has shown that, although a patient may not have a clinical sensitivity to an individual positive allergen at the time of the skin test, it is likely that, with repeated exposure, a clinical sensitivity will ultimately develop. Therefore, I include all positive reactors in my immunotherapy program.

PROCEDURES

Two principal approaches to immunotherapy are available to the veterinarian: a low-dose and a high-dose aqueous antigen schedule. The low-dose schedule is recommended for the novice allergist because it is less likely to cause adverse reactions. Its disadvantages, however, are that it takes much longer for clinical improvement to be seen, and it usually requires long-term maintenance therapy. In addition, even though most allergic animals have a high number of positive reactions, most laboratories do not like to prepare treatment vials containing more than 9 or 10 antigens. This is based partly on recommendations for humans, in whom reactions occur much more frequently. Allergists in human medicine are concerned, therefore, that their patients may receive too high an antigenic load with the resultant possibility of a severe adverse reaction. It is also based partly on the unproved belief that higher numbers of antigens do not provide as good a response to therapy. There is also a limit to the number of antigens at any given concentration that can physically be incorporated into 1 ml of extract. Therefore, a patient with large numbers of positive reactions may require multiple injection vials per treatment or several successive courses of treatment, to complete immunotherapy.

With the high-dose schedule, all skin-test-positive allergens can be easily divided into treatment groups of 5 to 7 allergens, to facilitate treatment. Clinical improvement usually occurs in a much shorter time, fewer injections are required, and, once the basic schedule is completed, maintenance therapy is generally not necessary. On average, it takes 9 to 12 weeks to complete the treatment schedule, with decided improvement often seen by about the fifth week of treatment. Dogs that have a good-to-excellent response may not require another injection once the initial series has been completed, whereas some require booster injections every few years, others every year, and still others several times a year. The procedure has the disadvantage, however, of being more likely to cause adverse reactions, some of which can be severe.

Low-Dose Therapy

Lose-dose custom treatment sets are supplied in either protein nitrogen units (PNUs) per ml or w/v. Unless otherwise specified, the total concentration per milliliter of antigens is divided by the number of antigens in the treatment vial. Therefore, if a 1000-PNU vial of extract contains 5 antigens, there will actually be only 200 PNU/ml of each antigen. If the vial has 10 antigens, there will only be 100 PNU/ml of each. The consequence of this type of therapy is obvious; treatment is inconsistent, the amount of antigen actually received may be too low to be of much value, and no two cases will necessarily be treated in the same manner. Consequently, the response rate, as well as the number and severity of possible adverse reactions, can vary.

Preparation of Treatment Sets

To maintain uniformity when prescribing or ordering treatment vials, specify the number of antigens to be included in each vial, as well as the number of units per milliliter of each antigen. Assume, therefore, that a 1000-PNU/ml treatment vial being prepared will contain 5 allergens, and a second vial will contain 8 allergens. If they are being prepared commercially, rather than from in-office stock concentrates, instructions to the manufacturer should clearly indicate that each vial is to contain 1000 PNU of **EACH** antigen, so the first vial will actually contain a total of 5000 PNU/ml, and the second vial will have a total of 8000 PNU/ml.

Treatment Schedule

Because no single injection procedure is used by all veterinary allergists, Table 11–1 is a composite of recommended schedules. Note the examples of three types of treatment sets, with one standardized in w/v and the other two in PNU. In spite of the different concentrations, all have been used successfully, and the choice is up to the individual veterinarian. If, however, the injections

Table 11–1. Suggested Concentrations and Dose Schedule for Low-Dose Immunotherapy

Injection No.	w/v PNU PNU	Vial No. 1 1:10,000 100/ml 200/ml (ml)	Vial No. 2 1:1000 1000/ml 2000/ml (ml)	Vial No. 3 1:100 10,000/ml 20,000/ml (ml)
1		0.1		
2		0.2		
3		0.4		
4		0.8		
5		1.0		
6			0.2	
7			0.4	
8			0.6	
9			0.8	
10			1.0	
11				0.2
12				0.3
13				0.4
14				0.5

MUST be given by the client, I suggest that the lowest concentration be dispensed, to minimize the possibility of adverse reactions.

Note also that there are three dosage levels, starting with the highest dilution (lowest concentration) and increasing in potency.

Injections are given weekly, but they can be increased to twice weekly, if necessary. Here again, no unanimity of opinion exists on whether to increase the dose with each injection during biweekly treatment or to increase the dose only on a weekly basis. Decisions are often made on a case-by-case basis, as experience is gained in treating patients.

Maintenance Therapy

Maintenance therapy is recommended with low-dose immunotherapy, based on the patient's response to the initial treatment schedule. If the response has been satisfactory, and the patient is comfortable at the time of the final injection, continue giving 0.5 ml of the highest concentration, beginning initially a week apart and gradually increasing the interval to a month apart. If the patient cannot be maintained on monthly injections without a recurrence of clinical signs, adjust the maintenance schedule for the maximum interval that will keep the patient comfortable. Schedules must be individualized for the specific patient because you may find that a pet that can be comfortable with monthly boosters during a period of low allergen load may require weekly injections during peak allergy periods. When the patient has been comfortable for a year or more, discontinue maintenance therapy to determine whether the patient still needs it. Should clinical signs occur, clinical remission may be obtained either by a single booster of the allergens present in the atmosphere at that time or by reinstitution of maintenance therapy. Depending on whether weeks or months have passed since the last maintenance dose, it may be necessary to administer a short course of stimulatory injections before resuming maintenance therapy.

Incomplete Response

If, on the other hand, the patient's improvement on completion of the initial series has been insufficient, do not stop at 0.5 ml followed by a maintenance schedule. Instead, continue to administer weekly or twice-weekly injections of the highest concentration, increasing the dose by 0.1 ml until a dose of 1.0 ml is reached. Depending on clinical response at this time, maintenance doses of 0.5 to 1.0 ml should be continued for several months, before increasing the time intervals.

The foregoing is to be viewed as a recommended schedule, not the only schedule. Dose recommendations have been extrapolated by different veterinarians, at different times, from procedures used in human med-

Table 11–2. Hypothetic High-Dose Treatment Groups

Group 1	Group 2	Group 3
Dust	Birch	Perennial rye grass
Feathers	Elm	Lamb's-quarter
Kapok	Maple	Marsh elder
Wool	Oak	English plantain
Ash	June grass	Ragweed

icine. Consequently, differing schedules are published in the veterinary literature. There is even a lack of uniformity in the human literature. Extensive clinical trials to determine optimal concentrations and dose schedules have not yet been conducted in the dog, so one cannot base a treatment regimen on scientifically objective data. Fortunately, such studies may not even be necessary because dogs seem to do so well on a purely empiric schedule.

High-Dose Therapy

High-dose therapy is not difficult to administer, but it can be complex to explain. To simplify the example, we will make a hypothetic assumption that a dog with 15 clear, positive skin-test reactions is to be treated. The antigens will be divided into groups, and the treatment schedule will be established.

Because high doses will be given, it is best not to include more than 5 or 6 allergens in any single treatment group, to minimize the possibility of adverse reactions. Therefore, the 15 allergens will be divided into 3 groups of 5 each. If necessary, up to 7, or even 8, antigens can be included in a single treatment group, depending on the total number of positive reactions.

To continue the example, let us assume that the positive reactions are to house dust, feathers, kapok, wool, ash, birch, elm, maple, oak, June grass, perennial rye, lamb's-quarters, marsh elder, English plantain, and ragweed. Although it is convenient to group them according to class, e.g., weed, grass, or environmental agent, they do not have to be grouped in any special order, so they will be arbitrarily combined as illustrated in Table 11–2.

Treatment Schedule

Three dose levels are administered for each group, allowing 1 to 3 weeks between the first

and second dose level for the same group, and 2 to 5 weeks between the second and third dose levels. Recent work in man suggests that 3 weeks between dose levels may be the most effective time interval, but this interval is apparently more optimal than critical.

The first, or base-level dose for each group contains 2000 PNU of each allergen in the group, for a total of 10,000 PNU in that group. The second dose level contains 4000 PNU of each allergen in the group, for a total of 20,000 PNU per group, whereas the third dose level contains 8000 PNU of each allergen for a total dose of 40,000 PNU. If, as noted previously, one must raise the number of antigens per treatment group to 7 or 8, it would naturally raise the total number of PNU per treatment because 2000, 4000, or 8000 units **PER ALLERGEN** would be still administered, regardless of the number of allergens included. Injection groups containing this number of allergens should be administered with caution and under close supervision.

To continue the hypothetic case example, Table 11–3 illustrates a typical schedule for a three-group series.

If there were four groups, the first dose of group four would be given as the seventh injection, the second dose would be given as the ninth injection, and the third dose would be given as the last injection.

The foregoing treatment schedule is based on many years of clinical experience, rather than on specific scientific data, and it has been an effective means of administering rapid immunotherapy. As an additional bonus, most dogs show improvement after the third or fourth injection, so it has the advan-

Table 11–3. Typical Immunotherapy Schedule for a Three-Group Series

Week 1	Dose level 1 of group 1
Week 2	Dose level 1 of group 2
Week 3	Dose level 1 of group 3
Week 4	Dose level 2 of group 1
Week 5	Dose level 2 of group 2
Week 6	Dose level 2 of group 3
Week 7	Dose level 3 of group 1
Week 8	Dose level 3 of group 2
Week 9	Dose level 3 of group 3

Dose level 1, 2000 PNU of *each* antigen in group
Dose level 2, 4000 PNU of *each* antigen in group
Dose level 3, 8000 PNU of *each* antigen in group

tage of indicating whether treatment will be effective. This situation is not true in all cases, however, because some dogs may not respond until the last injection and some may even need a few additional boosters.

Treatment Modification

Observations over the years have shown that the schedule can be modified without materially affecting the clinical outcome. The principal modification is to increase the frequency of injections at the lowest dose levels, in an attempt to shorten the total treatment time. This is of particular value when working with four or more groups of allergens. In such cases, injections of the lowest dose levels of **DIFFERENT** groups can be given as frequently as 3 days apart. The recommended time intervals for the second and third doses of the **SAME** group, however, should be followed as closely as possible. Moreover, scheduling difficulties may mandate lengthening the time between treatments. Such modifications in schedule do not reduce the effectiveness of treatment, but merely extend the time before clinical improvement is seen. When some portion of the schedule is modified, every effort should be made to return and adhere to the balance of the schedule as quickly as possible. The only other major reason for modifying the treatment schedule would be if there were adverse reactions. If such reactions cannot be controlled with antihistamines, as discussed later in this chapter, it would then be necessary to lower the dose, reduce the number of antigens in each treatment injection, or both. Figure 11–1 shows a favorable response to therapy in a dog with allergic dermatitis.

Alum-Precipitated Antigens

No chapter on immunotherapy would be complete without at least a brief discussion of alum-precipitated antigens. The first alum-precipitated preparation used in veterinary medicine, and probably still the best known, is a pyridine-extracted product mar-

keted under the trade name Allpyral (Hollister-Stier, West Haven, CT). It was my good fortune to do the first clinical studies on this product in veterinary medicine and to establish an acceptable dosage schedule for dogs.

Adsorption of the antigen onto alum slows down antigen release in the body and results in a slower, steadier immune stimulation. Its stimulatory effect lies somewhere between the rapidly absorbed aqueous and slowly released emulsion preparations.

To simplify dosage and administration, dilutions of stock concentrations are prepared so there are 500 PNU per ml of each allergen in a 10-ml vial. Starting with 50 PNU, rapidly increasing doses are given over gradually increasing time intervals, as shown in Table 11–4.

The same precautions must be followed with alum precipitates as with other extracts. During the years I used it, I never saw a generalized anaphylactic reaction, although occasional dogs developed milder reactions, such as generalized erythema, and one dog each developed mild urticaria and angioneurotic edema. The response to therapy was excellent and was usually evident by the third or fourth injection. My feeling over the years has been that it was more effective than aqueous extracts, with longer-lasting benefits.

The problem with recommending this product for general use is one of marketing, rather than efficacy. For a short time, the manufacturer of Allpyral aggressively entered the veterinary market, only to withdraw, leaving many veterinarians without treatment extracts for a short time. In addition, the number of available antigens is far smaller than for aqueous extracts, whereas the price is considerably higher. It is certainly worth trying, however, especially in animals with reactions to aqueous extracts.

ADVERSE REACTIONS

Whether low- or high-dose injection therapy is used, the potential for adverse reactions always exists. Although reactions are

Table 11–4. Alum-Precipitated Immunotherapy Schedule

Injection No.	1	2	3	4	5	6	7	8	9
Weeks	1	2	3	5	8	12	16	20	24
PNU	50	100	200	400	800	1500	3000	6000	10,000

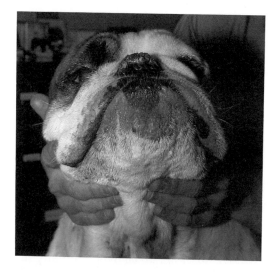 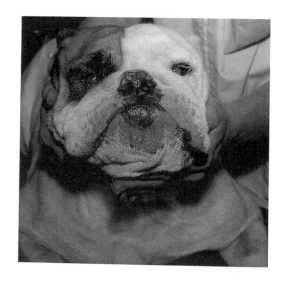

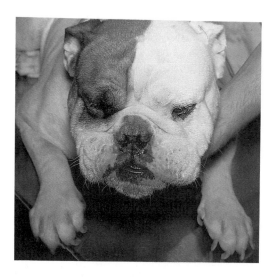

Fig. 11–1.   Seasonal allergic dermatitis in an English bull-dog during a course of immunotherapy. *A,* Condition before therapy. *B* and *C,* Visible improvements 1 and 2 months, respectively, after beginning therapy.

more likely to occur with high-dose therapy, severe, anaphylactoid reactions have even been reported following allergy skin testing, which certainly represents quantities of antigen far below those that would ever be administered therapeutically. Therefore, several precautions must be taken to minimize severe reactions or their consequences.

Prime among these is proper injection technique. **ALWAYS** apply negative pressure to the syringe to make sure that you are not in a blood vessel. If you see any trace of blood, redirect the needle and draw back on the plunger again.

Equally important, the patient should be kept in a treatment room, waiting room, or holding area for a minimum of 15 minutes following each injection treatment. Do not be lulled into a false sense of security because reactions have not occurred to prior injections. Although reactions can occur at any stage, the further into the injection series, the greater the potential for adverse reactions.

Finally, even though it is important to be prepared for reactions, they only occur in a small number of patients. In addition, most reactions are minor, not life-threatening, and they range from lethargy to increased pruritus, urticaria, and angioedema. Many of these reactions may not develop until several hours after the injection. On rare occasions, serum sickness-like reactions with depression and muscle stiffness have occurred several days after treatment. These reactions are not always easy to explain because they may not occur after subsequent injections, and patients often respond well to aspirin. I have only seen two deaths from acute anaphylaxis associated with immunotherapy. Although it was a disaster in those two cases, I do not consider it a problem statistically because it represents only two out of many thousands of injections. Both occurred following the last dose of the series, and in neither case did warning signs follow prior injections.

The development of adverse reactions does not mean that immunotherapy must be discontinued. They are warning signs, telling you to adjust the schedule. Several examples representing composites of actual histories illustrate the point.

Case No. 1

A patient undergoing immunotherapy has been responding favorably, when a sudden and marked increase in pruritus occurs following an injection. Does this represent a coincidental increase in the amount of allergen load triggering an increase in severity of clinical signs, or has the threshold of immunotherapy tolerance been exceeded? Checking pollen and mold counts with local hospitals or published reports gives information about atmospheric conditions. Questioning the patient's owner about the amount of outdoor activity during the previous week also supplies important information on which to base a decision. If the owner is unfortunate enough also to be allergic, questioning often reveals that both the pet and the owner had a concurrent increase in their allergic problem.

If all extraneous factors can be excluded, one may then reasonably assume that the injection dose has been too high. The strength of the dose should be reduced to the level of the last well-tolerated dose, maintained at that level for several injections, and then increased until the schedule is either completed or the top threshold tolerance dose is reached.

Alternatively, the scheduled doses can be continued, with a concurrent dose of 50 to 100 mg diphenhydramine given parenterally, depending on the severity of the reaction.

On rare occasions, severe pruritus continues in spite of dosage adjustments and re-quires a single injection of prednisolone or dexamethasone to break the reaction, after which immunotherapy can be continued using diphenhydramine, as described.

Case No. 2

A patient undergoing therapy suddenly develops urticaria or angioedema. Such reactions are acute and may be pruritic, but they are usually not life-threatening and generally look much worse than they really are, especially to the client.

The immediate reaction should be treated with epinephrine (discussed in more detail in case no. 3, later in this chapter) and parenteral diphenhydramine. Immunotherapy is continued, but the dosage should be reduced as previously discussed, and a concurrent dose of 100 mg parenteral diphenhydramine should be given with each injection. These patients generally do well, and treatment can usually be continued when proper precautions are taken.

When, on the other hand, the angioedema is accompanied by vomiting or diarrhea, the reaction is more serious because it suggests a splanchnic reaction and may represent a low-grade systemic anaphylactic response. Dosage should be cut by at least 50%, and additional injections must be given with extreme caution and must be preceded by parenteral diphenhydramine, given about 15 minutes before treatment. Patients must be watched for a minimum of 30 minutes following the injection, with epinephrine available for immediate injection, should the need arise.

All dogs with adverse reactions, regardless of the degree of severity, should receive oral diphenhydramine for the balance of the day. A possible additional measure in the more reactive patient is to administer 0.1 to 0.25 ml of sustained-release epinephrine (Sus-Phrine) just before the patient is released.

Case No. 3

The most serious reaction is anaphylaxis, characterized in the dog by sudden, severe vomiting, which is frequently hemorrhagic and can occur with or without diarrhea. In the cat, the reaction is usually respiratory, rather than splanchnic, and is characterized by severe pruritus of the face and ears, frantic rubbing with the feet, frothy nasal and oral discharge, and labored breathing. Both are acute anaphylactic reactions; they usually occur within 15 minutes, and both represent true medical emergencies.

The treatment of choice is parenteral epinephrine and diphenhydramine. Starting with an initial dose of 0.15 ml, a 1:1000 solution of aqueous epinephrine should be given subcutaneously, in small increments, until the patient is out of danger. At the same time, give 50 mg diphenhydramine intramuscularly. Continue to administer this dose of epinephrine every 10 minutes until the patient improves. At this point, reduce the dose of epinephrine to 0.1 ml every 15 minutes until the patient is out of danger or until a total of 1 ml epinephrine has been given. If the danger of relapse is suspected, 0.25 ml sustained-action epinephrine (Sus-Phrine) can be given for additional support.

Other supportive measures include maintenance of body temperature, oxygen inhalation, and fluid therapy. Corticosteroids are of little value in the treatment of the acute stage because they take too long to work. They may, however, be given to help prevent relapse.

Obviously, immunotherapy should be discontinued in these patients until newer, less reactive treatment allergens become available. Patients reactive to aqueous extracts may tolerate the slower-released alum-adsorbed allergens. If these allergens are used, however, proceed slowly and cautiously, until you are reasonably certain that no danger exists.

TREATMENT FAILURES

Because of the many reasons for treatment failure, a careful re-evaluation of the patient should be made, along with a review of the possibilities for failure. Chief among these are the following:

1. **Improper diagnosis.** Many conditions have clinical signs similar, if not identical, to allergy. Because some veterinarians often find it easier simply to label something an allergy, rather than to look for the correct diagnosis, a certain percentage of animals will inevitably not respond to allergy treatment because of misdiagnosis.

2. **Improper test performance or interpretation.** This error is not fatal; even experienced allergists make mistakes. Be aware of the human factor, however, and make every effort to avoid such errors.

3. **Insufficient test allergens or use of test mixtures.** Although I certainly do not advocate using maximum numbers of test antigens when first starting an allergy program, you should remember that the use of a limited number of antigens represents a SCREENING procedure, and occasional significant sensitivities are overlooked. Individual antigens in test mixtures, as discussed in Chapter 10, may be too dilute to elicit a reaction.

This limitation in no way minimizes the value of this testing, however, because a sufficient number of cases are still helped, and this reason, in itself, is enough to justify the procedure. Patients that do not respond can then be referred to a specialty practice.

4. **Use of low-potency or inactive antigens.** Both outdated and improperly stored extracts rapidly lose potency and cause poor skin-test results. Excessive temperatures inactivate the antigen, whereas freezing causes precipitation and loss of potency.

5. **Food allergy as a concurrent or exclusive diagnosis.** Food allergy, as discussed in Chapter 13, often cannot be differentiated from inhalant allergy and frequently accompanies it. Therefore, with any nonseasonal allergic problem, a food-allergy evaluation must be performed before initiating a skin-test and immunotherapy program.

6. **Failure to recognize concurrent medical problems or development of new ones following initial evaluation and immunotherapy.** Failure to do skin scrapings or to examine the skin closely for scabies or other ectoparasites constitutes a cardinal sin in veterinary allergy. These parasites are important contributory conditions in skin disease that necessitate multiple deep and shallow skin scrapings and the use of a flea comb. Nothing can be more irritating to the client, or more embarrassing to the veterinarian, than to complete a treatment series without improvement, only to find that the principal

problem was sarcoptic mange or some other parasite. Fleas are a common cause of treatment failure, so the patient's skin should be checked at every visit. If fleas or flea dirt are found, vigorous flea control should be instituted. Cheletiella, ticks, lice, and other ectoparasites are also occasional causes of pruritic skin disease. Hypothyroidism and other endocrine disturbances can cause alopecia and thin, dry skin, which can be pruritic.

7. **Failure to control environment conditions adequately.** Obviously, except for keeping allergic pets in an air-conditioned environment, little can be done about allergens in the atmosphere. Because the amount of control that can be imposed is so limited, one must direct one's efforts toward those conditions that can be controlled. Therefore, there is no justification for allowing an allergic pet to roll on the lawn, to root in the shrubbery beds, or to romp through piles of decaying leaves or compost heaps. During times of peak mold and pollen production, he should not run at will, he should be kept off lawns, and he should be walked along the driveway, or carried into the street, for his eliminations.

8. **Some patients, for reasons that are not understood, and in spite of proper diagnosis, positive skin-test results, and immunotherapy, fail to respond to treatment.** These patients represent serious treatment challenges because they often do not respond to medication and commonly become resistant to corticosteroids.

9. **Unidentified environmental allergens.** Every environment is uniquely individual and, although common threads may run through households, it is always possible that a patient may be allergic to a particular mold, dust, or other allergen that is found in higher concentration, or exclusively, in his home. Clients sometimes observe that the pet is better when in the hospital, the kennel, or when visiting friends in another household. When treatment fails, and you are secure in your diagnosis of allergy, it is often helpful to place the pet in the hospital for a 3- or 4-day observation period. The client should bring the food that the dog or cat has been eating regularly, so the only change is the environment. If improvement is sufficient,

the problem will probably be due to something within the household. The client is then instructed to place a clean bag in the vacuum cleaner and to collect dust from the floors, draperies, bedding, upholstered furniture, and other dust sources, for preparation of an autogenous dust extract. In addition, it can be helpful to place mold-collection plates around the house. If the molds that grow are different from those for which the pet was tested, stock or autogenous extracts should be obtained for both testing and treatment. Several of the companies manufacturing test and treatment allergens also prepare autogenous extracts, and they should be contacted for their specific collection procedures.

ECONOMIC CONSIDERATIONS

Bulk allergenic extracts can be expensive, and until you have developed an allergy practice large enough to merit an investment of several thousand dollars, it would make more sense to purchase skin-testing antigens only and to order individual prescription treatment allergens for each case. The disadvantage of this procedure is that it can take up to 5 weeks to receive the extracts because they must be compounded, standardized, and tested for sterility before they can be shipped. On the other hand, you do not have a major investment in materials that may become outdated before you use them.

When ordering custom treatment extracts, be sure to have the client prepay the cost of the extracts before you order them. Otherwise, he may change his mind, or may not show up to start the treatment series, and you may have to pay for extracts that cannot be used.

CONCURRENT USE OF STEROIDS AND OTHER MEDICATIONS

Considerable controversy has arisen over the years over whether corticosteroids interfere with the tolerogenic response to immunotherapy or, for that matter, the development of immunity through vaccinations and other biologic therapy. Although steroids and other medical therapies are discussed in Chapter 12, some comments about their use are pertinent at this time. Corticosteroids do not seem to interfere with allergy skin tests in man, and before the advent of inhalant corticosteroids, it was not unusual for allergists to use them systemically for the control of severe asthma, even while patients were undergoing immunotherapy. Extrapolating from past human experience, many veterinary dermatologists do not hesitate to use these drugs in patients undergoing allergy injection therapy, even though the limited studies reported in the veterinary literature are contradictory, and there have been no studies demonstrating that interference does not occur in the dog or cat during immunotherapy for allergy.

Corticosteroids

Based on the biologic activity of corticosteroids, these drugs are contraindicated during immunotherapy and have little to commend their use, except for the temporary relief of clinical signs. The most serious concern is their effect on both lymphocytes and humoral antibody. In the dog, there is dramatic drop in total circulating lymphocytes that may continue for long periods after treatment has stopped. I have followed serial blood samples in dogs in which lymphocyte counts did not return to normal for almost 6 months. Because blocking antibody is produced by lymphocytes, it stands to reason that the probability of a favorable response would be diminished.

In addition, steroids have a direct effect on circulating antibody itself. In postrabies vaccination studies, for example, circulating antibody levels dropped markedly following administration of corticosteroids.[1] Therefore, my standard recommendation, at this time, is to **AVOID THEIR USE** during biologic therapy.

Antihistamines and Other Anti-inflammatory Agents

On the other hand, antihistamines, aspirin, and nonsteroidal anti-inflammatory agents can be used with impunity during **treatment.** Because these agents have no direct effect on the development of the immune response, there is no reason they cannot be used during immunotherapy.

REFERENCE

1. Soave, O., and Fuenzalida, E.: Effect of cortisone on antibody level of mice given rabies antigens three months earlier. Am. J. Vet. Res., *30*:643, 1969.

12 ‖ *Medical Management of Allergic Disease*

Objectively, the ideal way to manage allergic disease is to identify the offending allergen(s) and to avoid or eliminate them. Except for food, however, avoidance is generally difficult, if not impossible, necessitating other means of control. The most viable alternative is immunotherapy, in which the immune system is changed so as to render the patient incapable of reacting adversely following exposure to allergens. Yet immunotherapy is sometimes impossible or impractical, so medical therapy becomes the treatment of choice, as either supportive or substitute therapy.

INDICATIONS

The principal indications for medical therapy are as follows:

1. **For short-term, temporary relief while waiting to start immunotherapy.** Unless treatment antigens are prepared in the office, several weeks can elapse between skin testing and receipt of extracts from commercial laboratories. Therefore, to keep the patient comfortable during the waiting period, medical therapy can provide excellent relief without interfering with the induction of the immune response.

2. **As an adjunct to biologic therapy.** Nonsteroidal medical therapy can help to keep the patient comfortable until immunotherapy takes effect.

3. **For relief of the transient recurrence of an allergic attack.** Even patients with the best-controlled allergies can have occasional periods of discomfort, which can usually be reversed with medication. If the problem is severe enough to require booster injections, medication will often afford a measure of relief until an appointment can be made for the injection.

4. **Sometimes allergy skin testing and immunotherapy are neither practical nor realistic.** These circumstances include older dogs (arbitrarily, over 13 years old) whose anticipated life expectancy is too short to benefit fully from injection therapy and clients who are either unable or unwilling to complete an immunotherapy program.

5. **Finally, some patients are unable to tolerate even the smallest doses of immunotherapy.** Rather than risk serious, or even fatal, reactions, medical management becomes the treatment of choice.

The principal classes of therapeutic agents useful in the medical management of allergic disease are corticosteroids, antihistamines, and nonsteroidal anti-inflammatory agents. In addition, histamine antagonists, antiserotonin agents, immunosuppressive agents, and other miscellaneous drugs also occasionally play a useful role.

CORTICOSTEROIDS

The most commonly used, and most often abused, drugs for the treatment of allergy are the corticosteroids. Because they work well initially, they are often used in lieu of a definitive diagnosis. Unfortunately, most of the serious side effects of these drugs are insidious and thereby promote continuous use, ultimately leading to long-term corticosteroid abuse. In addition, the obvious side effects, polydipsia, polyuria, and polyphagia, have become so commonplace to the veterinarian as virtually to have lost meaning. Even worse, many patients receive long-term therapy without adequate supervision and therefore suffer more from acquired serious corticosteriod side effects than from the initial problem for which they were treated.

Specific Effects

Corticosteroids can have deep and profound effects on almost every system. They either directly or indirectly affect the following:

1. Carbohydrate metabolism

2. Protein metabolism
3. Water and electrolyte balance
4. The endocrine system
5. The musculoskeletal system
6. Inflammatory reactions
7. The hematopoietic system
8. Antibody production
9. Mood and behavior

Carbohydrate Metabolism

Corticosteroids increase gluconeogenesis and decrease peripheral glucose use. This process leads to increased tissue glycogen stores, particularly in the liver. As gluconeogenesis increases, hyperglycemia and glucosuria may develop and, in turn, may aggravate existing diabetes mellitus or may even activate an incipient diabetic state.

Protein Metabolism

Protein catabolism is increased, whereas protein anabolism is inhibited. Decreased anabolism can depress growth in the young and may inhibit or delay wound healing, with weak incision lines following surgery. Moreover, corticosteroids may inhibit antibody production and even lead to loss of preformed immunoglobulins, especially during long-term therapy or following the use of such long-acting agents as betamethasone.

Water and Electrolyte Metabolism

Sodium retention and potassium diuresis are common sequelae of corticosteroid therapy and can lead to edema, hypokalemia, muscle weakness, hypochloremia, and metabolic acidosis. These changes can be relieved with potassium therapy and can usually be prevented by giving potassium chloride or by feeding the patient potassium-rich foods, such as bananas and orange juice.

Endocrine System

Prolonged corticosteroid therapy lowers circulating thyroxine (T_4) levels and can reduce, or even suppress adrenocorticotropic hormone (ACTH) production because of its effect on the hypothalamic-pituitary-adrenal axis.

Musculoskeletal System

Patients may develop osteoporosis, because of the inhibitory effect of corticosteroids on both calcium absorption from the gut and osteogenesis. The protein catabolic effect already discussed results in laxity, flaccidity, and weakness of tendons, ligaments, and muscles. The flaccidity and thinning of the abdominal muscles give the patient the potbellied appearance typical of canine Cushing's disease.

Anti-inflammatory Action

The exact mechanism of action of corticosteroids is unknown, but much of this effect is believed to be due to a decrease in both fibroblast activity and granuloma formation. This is a double-edged sword because, although this effect reduces pain and discomfort, it also reduces the tissue's ability to wall off and contain infections and foreign bodies.

Steroids also apparently stabilize lysosomal membranes in damaged tissues and thereby inhibit or reduce the release of digestive enzymes. Again, although this effect helps to reduce inflammation, it also interferes with the normal cleanup processes in affected tissues.

In addition, corticosteroids may possibly inhibit prostaglandin formation, further reducing inflammation.

Hematopoietic Effects and Antibody Production

The most obvious effects on the hematologic system are a reduction in circulating eosinophils, lymphopenia, involution of lymphoid tissue, and neutrophilia. The effect on the lymphoid system obviously affects antibody production, which is reduced. As mentioned before, previously formed antibody may even be lost following steroid therapy. Therefore, one should neither vaccinate patients receiving long-term steroid therapy nor administer a long-acting steroid concurrently with a vaccine.

Mood and Behavior

Both euphoria and depression may occur. In man, depression can become severe enough to lead to suicide. Aggressive behavior has also been seen in both man and animals. I once treated a golden retriever with a marvelous temperament that became extremely aggressive and difficult to handle following corticosteroid administration. On withdrawal of the medication, his normally sweet disposition returned. The owner, a physician, was particularly intrigued by this behavioral response. He himself had developed asthma while in medical school and was given steroid therapy. Within a short time, his classmates noted a startling, aggressive change in his normal, jovial behavior that lasted until the steroid was withdrawn.

Serum Chemistries

Even small doses of steroids can have a profound effect on clinical chemistries. Liver enzymes are particularly affected, as evidenced by lipemia and highly elevated levels of alkaline phosphatase, serum glutamic-pyruvic transaminase (SGPT), and gamma-glutamyl transpeptidase (GGTP). The alkaline phosphatase level may be high enough to take months to return to normal following withdrawal of the steroid. Hyperglycemia may also be associated with treatment.

How Glucocorticoids Work in Allergic Disease

No one is certain exactly how corticosteroids work to relieve allergic disease, although over the years the pieces of the puzzle have been slowly falling into place and will be discussed briefly in this chapter. In general, their anti-inflammatory effect plays a significant role in alleviating much of the irritation and pruritus associated with allergic skin disease. By inhibiting vasodilation and increased vascular permeability, these drugs reduce much of the edema associated with allergic inflammation.

Moreover, it is believed that steroids in some way stabilize the mast cell wall, thereby reducing or preventing degranulation and the release of inflammatory mediators. When these agents inhibit the release of lysosomal enzymes, as noted previously, antigen processing by macrophages does not proceed properly, and the normal progression of antigen/antibody reactions is impeded. Inherent in the control of inflammatory mediators is the ability of corticosteroids to form lipocorten, which interferes with

phospholipase activity, thereby blocking the arachidonic acid cascade and preventing the conversion of phospholipids to leukotrienes and prostaglandins. Evidence also suggests that steroids may block the action of inflammatory mediators on the target cells themselves.

Preferred Agents and Methods of Use

To minimize the possibility of undesirable side effects, one should use alternate-day therapy whenever possible and short-acting steroids at all times at the lowest dose that produces a therapeutic effect. Nothing is more distressing than to watch an adverse reaction develop and to be unable to do anything about it because the drug administered will stay in the patient's system for a long time.

Prednisone and prednisolone are the drugs of choice; their short half-lives make them ideally suited for alternate-day therapy. Of the two, prednisolone is preferred because it is the active form of the drug. Prednisone must be converted to prednisolone in the liver, and because glucocorticoids alter liver enzymes and produce abnormal liver enzyme profiles, one cannot preclude the possibility of liver changes sufficient to interfere with the conversion of prednisone. Therefore, it seems reasonable to use the active form and to forego the necessity for liver transformation.

When long-term therapy cannot be avoided, one must institute alternate-day therapy as soon after stabilization of the condition as possible. To do this, determine the lowest daily dose of prednisolone that will still render clinical control of the allergy. The dose is then doubled and is given every other day. If control is still maintained, the dose should be gradually reduced until one finds the lowest dose still capable of maintaining the patient in comfort. This then becomes the maintenance dose for as long as steroid therapy is needed.

When short-term therapy with a longer-lasting effect is needed, dexamethasone may be used. This drug should not be used for long-term maintenance therapy, and it cannot be used orally for alternate-day therapy, however, because of its long-life, relative to prednisolone. In theory, a short-acting steroid given in the morning clears the serum quickly enough for ACTH still to be released on the evening of the day the steroid is given. Cortisol released on the following day helps to maintain the steroid's effect. Even though total cortisol levels are lower without exogenous steroid administration, the level of cortisol is usually sufficient to control the inflammatory reaction. The following day, exogenous steroid is again administered, and the cycle continues. Studies have shown that steroids given in this manner produce less adrenal suppression than when the drugs are given daily. Because longer-acting steroids take considerably longer to clear the serum, even alternate-day therapy does not prevent adrenal suppression.

Guidelines for steroid therapy include the following:

1. Always use the smallest effective dose.
2. Avoid extra-long-acting and repository types.
3. **Taper the dose. Do not stop abruptly** unless the steroid has only been used for a few days.
4. Avoid long-term therapy in allergic disorders, unless absolutely necessary, in which case use alternate-day therapy.
5. Do not perform allergy skin tests until sufficient time has elapsed following steroid withdrawal.
6. During long-term therapy, the patient should be monitored carefully for evidence of hypokalemia, bone decalcification, loss of collagen, thinning of skin with hair loss, adrenal hypoplasia, and iatrogenic Cushingoid and Addisonian signs (if the steroid is withdrawn too rapidly).
7. Perform regular blood counts, differential counts, and serum chemistry profiles, so that adjustments can be made to medication schedules, if necessary, and to maintain baseline reference data in the event of an emergency.

ANTIHISTAMINES

Antihistamines alone are of limited value in the treatment of allergic disease, although they are occasionally very effective. To understand how antihistamines work, as well as why they often fail, it is important briefly to review the mediators of allergic inflammation. Because a detailed discussion of this fascinating subject is beyond the purview of this text, I refer the reader to Tizard's *Veterinary Immunology* or any human allergy or immunology text.

The principal mediators in the dog, and presumably the cat, are histamine, prostaglandins, thromboxanes, leukotrienes (formerly known as SRS-A, the slow-reacting substance of anaphylaxis), and kinins. To these substances must be added a host of contributory mediators, such as several chemotactic factors, complement, thrombocyte factors, and others that enter into inflammatory reactions. Although some patients respond well to antihistamines, it becomes quickly obvious that a maximal response should not be expected, unless one administers additional therapeutic agents capable of counteracting other inflammatory mediators.

Following mast-cell degranulation and mediator release, histamine binds to specific histamine (H_1) receptor sites, initiating its specific pharmacologic effects, such as vasodilation, increased capillary permeability with edema, contraction of nonvascular smooth muscle, and stimulation of sensory nerve endings, with itching.

The chemical configuration of antihistamines is such that its structure "fits" the H_1 receptor site, blocks histamine, and prevents the adverse reaction. The aim of therapy therefore is to flood the receptor sites with enough antihistamine to "cover" as many open receptors as possible. This approach precludes intermittent therapy because histamine has a much stronger affinity for the receptor sites than most antihistamines and is not replaced once attached. In fact, if the allergic reaction is severe enough, and if sufficient histamine is released, it may displace the antihistamine. Newer antihistamines are now being developed, however, that will overcome this problem, in that they bind so tightly to the H_1 receptor that they either cannot be displaced by histamine or remain attached in situ for long periods of time. Although these agents are not yet available in the United States, experimental studies in the dog and clinical experience in man in

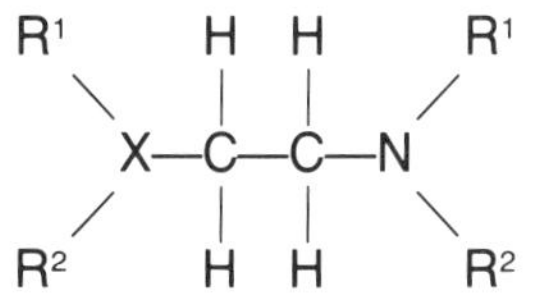

$$R^1 \quad H \quad H \quad R^1$$
$$X—C—C—N$$
$$R^2 \quad H \quad H \quad R^2$$

Fig. 12–1.   Basic ethylamine antihistamine structure.

other countries has been encouraging. Because of the strong affinity of the newer antihistamines for H_1 receptors, they also have the obvious advantage of only requiring once-daily administration.

In addition to the H_1 receptors for histamine are the H_2 receptors, which also seem to play a role in allergic inflammation. Unlike lung tissue, in which H_1 and H_2 receptors apparently modulate each other, H_2 receptors in skin blood vessels seem to have a complementary effect. Although H_2 receptors are less numerous than H_1, some evidence shows that when H_2 blockers are used in conjunction with H_1 antihistamines, one sees an apparent, small, but measurable, improvement over that gained by the use of antihistamines alone.

H_1 Blockers

The basic structure of most antihistamines is a substituted ethylamine, as shown in Figure 12–1.

Substitutions at the X position change the compound, so by substituting the X with an oxygen, it becomes an aminoalkyl ether; if displaced by nitrogen, it is an ethylenediamine compound, and carbon changes it to an alkylamine. By manipulating the structure, one may alter and change its relative pharmacologic activity and side effects (Table 12–1).

Table 12–1 is only a sample of available antihistamines and represents those with which I have had clinical experience. Most of these agents have been available for many years, so a background of experience has developed relative to their safety and efficacy.

The substituted ethylamines represent the largest group of generally recognized antihistamines. They are usually similar in activity, but differ in the intensity of their side effects.

Terfenadine (Seldane) represents an entirely new class of compounds, and although I am not overly impressed with its efficacy, other veterinarians have reported good results.

Hydroxyzine (Atarax) has both antihistamine and tranquilizing effects that have been beneficial for some patients. In particular, the drug promotes relaxation and mild sedation, which, when combined with the drug's histamine-antagonizing effects, have helped to relieve many patients.

Cyproheptadine (Periactin) differs in that, in addition to its antihistamine action, it also acts as an antiserotonin agent. Antiserotonin agents are discussed in more detail later in this chapter.

Azatadine maleate (Optimine) is also a methylpiperidine compound related to cyproheptidine with antihistamine, antiserotonin, anticholinergic, and sedative properties. I have had limited experience with this drug, but as with terfenadine, I am not overly impressed with its efficacy and, except for its b.i.d. dosage, see no advantage in using this drug over much less expensive antihistamines. It may be more effective when combined with other classes of antihistamines, but this must await further clinical trial.

Doxepin HCl is a tricyclic antidepressant drug that has been used at a dose of 1 to 2 mg/kg. Although I have not yet used this drug on my patients, other veterinarians have reported favorably on its use. Its effect seems to be related to its phenothiazine-related structure and its subsequent antihistamine and anticholinergic action. It is a particularly potent H_1 and H_2 blocker.

Although most antihistamines have a wide margin of safety, they are not innocuous and can have significant side effects, including sedation, gastrointestinal disturbances, allergic reactions, teratogenicity, hyperexcitability, and even convulsions. The principal side effect, sedation, is of little concern because pets do not have to drive, work, or handle dangerous machinery. In fact, the sedative effect is beneficial; it helps the patient to rest and reduces self-mutilation. These drugs should not be given to pregnant dogs or to dogs being bred because of the reported teratogenicity of these agents.

If one antihistamine does not work, try an-

Table 12–1. Representative Preparations and Dosages of Antihistamines Useful in Small Animal Medicine

Class and Generic Name	Trade Name	Dose (mg)	Parenteral Available
Ethanolamines			
Diphenhydramine	Benadryl	25–50 t.i.d.	yes
Ethylenediamines			
Tripelennamine	Pyribenzamine	25–50 t.i.d.	yes
Pyrilamine maleate	Triaminic (with decongestant)	25–50 t.i.d.	
Alkylamines			
Chlorpheniramine	Chlor-Trimeton	4 q.i.d	yes
Piperazines			
Hydroxyzine	Atarax	10–50 t.i.d.	yes
Phenothiazines			
Promethazine	Phenergan	25 t.i.d.	yes
Trimeprazine	Temaril	5-mg Spansules t.i.d.	
Methylpiperidine			
Cyproheptadine	Periactin	4 t.i.d.–q.i.d.	
Azatadine maleate	Optimine	1–2 b.i.d.	
Terfenadine	Seldane	60 q. 12 h.	

other. Even though they all work in similar fashion, they may have different affinities for receptor sites or even for certain receptor sites. If you are not satisfied with the clinical response after trying a few different agents, try combining antihistamines of different chemical classes; this will frequently give a better response. There are no firm rules for combined antihistamine dosages, but I have used the full dose for each antihistamine with no apparent serious side effects.

Finally, it is often necessary to increase the dose beyond that generally recommended. This increase is usually not a problem because of the wide margin of safety of most antihistamines. However, it is important to remember that both side effects and toxicity can occur, and the client should be warned to keep the patient under general observation and to report any unusual signs. One must become familiar with the pharmacology and side effect of antihistamines prescribed, to enable the client both to be properly advised and to anticipate potential problems.

An effective way to initiate antihistamine therapy in animals, especially when the condition is severe and unlikely to respond to antihistamine therapy alone, is to use short-term combined antihistamine/corticosteroid therapy. The steroid dose is rapidly tapered and discontinued, whereas the antihistamine is maintained at full dosage. If the antihistamine is reduced in dose or stopped, clinical signs will usually return and will generally not respond to reinstitution of antihistamine therapy alone. When such a situation occurs, the entire process must be repeated, using both corticosteroids and antihistamines to reinstitute therapy.

H_2 Blockers

The two best known H_2 blockers are cimetidine (Tagamet) and ranitidine (Zantac). In allergic diseases, neither their value nor specific dosages have been established at this time. Because both H_1 and H_2 receptors seem to be involved in allergic dermatitis, however, these drugs would be worth trying in combination with other antihistamines. The suggested dose of ranitidine is 2.2 to 4.4 mg/kg orally every 12 hours; that of cimetidine is 5 to 10 mg/kg every 6 to 12 hours. These doses are extrapolated from those recommended for the treatment of gastric problems in the dog.

ANTIBIOTICS

Antibiotics often improve the pruritus and inflammation associated with allergic skin disease, although why they work is sometimes uncertain. Atopic skin disease is often accompanied by a secondary, superficial infection that can, at times, be pruritic. Moreover, the bacteria found in pyoderma or other skin infections can sometimes induce a pruritic hypersensitivity reaction. In either case,

Table 12–2. Useful Antibiotics in Atopic Inflammation and Pruritus

Antibiotic	Suggested Dose (mg/lb)
Cephalexin (Keflex)	12–15 b.i.d.
Cefadroxil (Cefa Tabs)	10 b.i.d.
Cephadrine (Velosef)	12–25 b.i.d.
Oxacillin (Prostaphlin)	6 t.i.d. or q.i.d.
Chloramphenicol (Chloromycetin)	25 t.i.d.
Sulfamethoxizole-trimethoprim (Septra, Bactrim)	10–15 b.i.d.
Amoxicillin/clavulanate K (Clavamox, Augmentin)	6.25 b.i.d.
Lincomycin (Lincocin)*	8–10 t.i.d.

*Although lincomycin is a popular antibiotic among many veterinary clinicians, I have not found it particularly useful in patients that I treat for skin disease. Because lincomycin is often used as a first-line antibiotic, the bacteria may have become resistant to the drug by the time I see these patients as referral cases.

antibiotic therapy would be indicated. In fact, atopic animals that fail to respond adequately to immunotherapy often benefit from a course of antibiotics.

Antibiotics should be selected on the basis of their known benefit in skin disease, the animal's tolerance to the medication, ease of administration, and cost. I have often wondered whether cephalexin has a specific antipruritic action because, shortly after it became generally available, many clients began to report that it seemed to be effective in reducing pruritus, even before an appreciable reduction in inflammation was seen. Since then, the cephalosporins have been my drug of choice in atopic skin disease and pyoderma. A list of useful antibiotics and their suggested dosages is found in Table 12–2.

ANTISEROTONIN COMPOUNDS

Serotonin antagonists represent a uniquely effective, yet puzzling class of compounds for the treatment of allergic disease. Although serotonin, along with histamine and heparin, are important inflammatory mediators in the rodent, they either play no such role, or are considered of no significance, in man, dog, or cat. Yet in a series of investigative trials I conducted many years ago, with a variety of different antiserotonin compounds, these drugs were as effective as glucocorticoids, whether given orally, parenterally, or topically. They even had the same side effects, but with a difference. In addition

to polydipsia, polyuria, and polyphagia, many of these dogs also hallucinated, snapping at imaginary flying objects, staring off into space, and barking at the moon for hours on end.

Only three preparations currently available have antiserotonin activity: methysergide maleate tablets (Sansert), cyproheptadine (Periactin) and azatadine maleate (Optimine). Of these, methysergide is the most effective, but also the most likely to cause undesirable reactions.

The dose for methysergide is 2 mg 2 to 3 times daily. Before using it, however, one should become familiar with its listed side effects in man. No serious complications were seen in dogs with the use of these compounds during the investigative trial, but this does not mean they cannot occur.

Cyproheptadine and azatadine are excellent drugs to try because they have both antihistaminic and antiserotonin properties. The dose is 4 mg t.i.d. for cyproheptadine and 1 to 2 mg b.i.d. for azatadine, and they may be combined with other antihistamines.

ANTIPROSTAGLANDINS

Prostaglandins are a complex family of lipid compounds, many of which are derived from cell-wall phospholipids via the arachidonic acid cascade. Some members of the family have potent inflammatory capabilities. In addition to the better known prostaglandins E and F (PGE and PGF), prostaglandins also include the thromboxanes (Tx) and prostacyclins (PGI). They are widely distributed throughout the body and enter into most inflammatory reactions. Inflamed skin has a marked increase in prostaglandin content, justifying the use of both oral and topical prostaglandin antagonists as possible adjunctive therapy for allergic disease.

Aspirin

The principal antiprostaglandin compounds are aspirin and indomethacin. Because aspirin is poorly tolerated by many dogs and may cause vomiting, one should administer it as either a buffered tablet or combined with an antacid. It can be toxic for cats and should be avoided in this species. Depending on the animal's size, the dose is

2.5 to 5 gr. (150 to 300 mg) t.i.d. Acetaminophen (Tylenol) is **not** a substitute for aspirin, which is used for its specific antiprostaglandin/anti-inflammatory activity. Acetaminophen has no such activity.

When using aspirin in allergic disease, however, some evidence indicates that aspirin can actually increase the production of inflammatory mediators. Therefore, if aspirin is used, and if no beneficial effect is noted or the patient worsens, it should be discontinued.

Aspirin has also been reported of value in the prevention of food allergy and pseudoallergy. Its mechanism of action for this use is unknown, but it may interfere in some way with the induction of the reaction.

Triethanolamine Salicylate

Triethanolamine salicylate (Aspercreme), available as both a topical lotion and a cream, has some antiprostaglandin activity that may be helpful in some dogs by locally counteracting prostaglandin in inflamed skin. As with all topicals, the dog must be kept occupied for at least 20 minutes after application, to prevent licking, and the drug should not be used on cats. To date, clinical response has been equivocal.

Indomethacin

Indomethacin has been tried in dogs, but no safe dose is recognized, and it should only be used when all other therapies have failed. Because of the potential for severe, serious side effects, the smallest effective dose should be used, and the patient **MUST BE** monitored carefully.

PHYSIOLOGIC HISTAMINE ANTAGONISTS

These agents differ from antihistamines in that they antagonize the physiologic effects of histamine, rather than blocking the action of histamine at the cell receptor site. The principal antagonists available for use in small animal medicine are the sympathomimetic drugs ephedrine sulfate and the xanthines, theophylline and aminophylline. Although their major effects are the induction of bronchodilation and smooth muscle relax-

ation, they may also be of some value as adjunctive therapy in allergic inhalant disease.

Ephedrine

Ephedrine, derived from the ma huang (ephedra) plant, is administered orally in doses of 10 to 25 mg t.i.d., depending on the size of the patient and the response to treatment. Because ephedrine is most useful as a bronchial smooth muscle relaxant, its greatest value is in the treatment of asthma and asthmatic bronchitis. It can be beneficial in the treatment of allergic inhalant disease when given with antihistamines or other mediator antagonists, however.

Xanthines

To understand how theophylline (methylxanthine) and aminophylline (theophylline ethylenediamine) may possibly help to control allergic reactions, we must briefly review the cAMP/cGMP system, or so-called second messenger system of mast cells. Cyclic adenosine monophosphate (cAMP) and cyclic guanosine monophosphate (cGMP) are, in a sense, the yin and yang of many cellular functions, each exerting a regulatory effect on the other. Following antigen coupling of immunoglobulin E (IgE) antibodies on mast cells, changes occur (the first messenger) that initiate the chain of events ultimately resulting in degranulation and mediator release (the third messenger). Between these two events, within the cell, lies the cAMP/cGMP second messenger system. Anything that raises the AMP level or reduces the GMP level inhibits degranulation. Conversely, raising GMP levels or lowering AMP levels increases degranulation and release of mediators.

Theophylline and aminophylline are believed to increase AMP levels, thereby helping to reduce the amount of mediator release. Although their most effective use is bronchodilatory, they are occasionally of value as adjunctive therapy with other pharmacologic agents. A dose of 100 to 200 mg t.i.d., depending on the animal's size, is usually sufficient. Sustained-action products, such as Theo-Dur, can be given twice daily at the same dose.

SODIUM CROMOGLYCATE

Sodium cromoglycate appears to have a direct effect on the mast cell, apparently by stabilizing it and inhibiting mediator release. Unfortunately, at the present time, only the ophthalmic solution appears to be clinically useful for dogs; it has been beneficial in the treatment of allergic conjunctivitis at a dose of one drop in each eye q.i.d.

Sodium cromoglycate is not indicated for the relief of acute allergic states, in that it takes several days before a response is seen. Therefore, it must be used regularly and consistently if the allergic condition is to be controlled. The most widely used form in man is an inhalant powder or solution for use in the prevention and treatment of asthma. An injectable solution tried experimentally in dogs was found to be very toxic. An oral form not yet available in this country has been effective in the treatment of food allergy. Because this is a first-generation drug, one hopes that modifications of later generations will prove clinically useful in animals, as well as in people.

SOAKS AND RINSES

Although I rarely recommend shampoos or baths for allergic skin conditions, I have found that soaks and rinses are often of value. Plain cool-water baths, in particular, can be soothing, providing relief for hours in some otherwise intractable pruritic states.

Aveeno Colloidal Oatmeal Bath

Aveeno bath is composed of colloidal oatmeal without soaps or synthetic detergents. The adsorptive properties of oatmeal cleanse and soothe the skin, often providing relief for several days. It is available in both regular and oilated forms, for dogs with dry skins. The adsorptive qualities of oatmeal are well known, and I have recommended the use of oatmeal flakes as a dry cleanser, rubbed into the coat and then brushed thoroughly, for over 35 years.

One to two tablespoons of the Aveeno powder are mixed with cool water. The coat is soaked thoroughly with this mixture, either by sponging it onto the coat or, if the pet is small enough, by soaking the pet in a tub or basin. I have used this preparation for many years, and although it is sometimes messy, with an odor that some people find unpleasant, I have rarely had complaints because of the relief afforded the pet following its use.

Medicated Hydrotherapy

Because secondary infection generally accompanies most allergic seborrheas, medicated soaks using "tamed" organic iodine or chlorhexidine can afford excellent relief. Whether because of the stimulation of the skin produced by the hydrotherapy jets or because of the improved penetration of the antibacterial agent into the skin, when the agent is administered in a whirlpool the effect appears to be significantly enhanced.

Oil Rinses

Humectants and oil rinses applied to the skin are also often beneficial. They work by humidifying the skin and counteracting water loss, thus helping to keep the skin from drying out and becoming even more itchy.

MISCELLANEOUS SUPPORTIVE AGENTS

Vitamin C

High-dose vitamin C therapy is a controversial modality in human medicine, having been used by some allergists since its discovery, with little more than a clinical impression that it was beneficial. With this as background, a limited number of uncontrolled clinical studies reported favorable results following the use of high-dose therapy in cases of human pollinosis. Even though the dog manufactures its own vitamin C, and supplementation is generally not considered necessary, I conducted a clinical trial many years ago to see whether it might be of value anyway. In the protocol established, a group of seasonally allergic dogs were given 500 mg vitamin C throughout the year. Five weeks before the start of the weed allergy season, the dose was increased to 2000 mg, and maintained at that level until the end of the season, when the dose was again reduced to 500 mg. In spite of a severe allergy season that year, about half the dogs remained comfortable. When vitamin C was withheld the following year, all the dogs developed clinical signs. When therapy was reinstituted, improvement was again seen and continued throughout the follow-up period. Admittedly, this study must be considered anecdotal because it was not a double-blind or double-blind-crossover study. Vitamin C has been used on difficult cases since then, however, and occasional dogs have had a good response.

We do not know exactly how vitamin C works in helping to control allergy. One theory suggests that it enters into cyclic nucleotide reactions, increasing the levels of AMP or reducing those of GMP. Significant factors are that ascorbic acid therapy is inexpensive, it rarely causes problems except unusual urinary crystal formation, and excess vitamin not used by the body is simply excreted. Therefore, it is worth trying at a daily dose of 1500 to 2000 mg orally.

EPA and Other Fatty Acid Therapy

In recent years, researchers have become interested in the possibility of interrupting, or modifying, the arachidonic acid cascade through the use of eicosapentanoic acid (EPA), derived from fish oil, linoleic acid, and gamma-linolenic acids. During inflammatory skin reactions, phospholipases act on cell membranes to release phospholipids, including arachidonic acid, which is metabolized either by cyclo-oxygenase into prostaglandins, prostacyclins, or thromboxanes, or by lipoxygenases into leukotrienes.

Theoretically, if patients' diets are rich in EPA, gamma-linolenic acid, or linoleic acid, the structures of these acids will be such that they will be either incorporated into the cell wall (EPA) and compete with arachidonic acid for lipo-oxygenase and cyclo-oxygenase or, in the case of linoleic and gamma-linolenic acid, metabolized to products that will block the transformation of arachidonic acid to inflammatory leukotrienes and one of the prostaglandin series. By competing for, and thereby "consuming," these metabolic enzymes, less arachidonic acid will be metabolized and less inflammatory mediators will be produced.

Unfortunately, although the theory is sound, reality is such that only about 20% of patients actually derive any real benefit from the treatment. In treating allergic inflammation, however, in which every positive response is a plus, even a 20% success rate justifies a trial with these fatty acids as adjunctive therapy.

Immunosuppressive Agents

Because of their toxicity and side effects, these agents are rarely used, but occasional reports of therapeutic success appear in the human literature. For example, at least one paper describes the use of 5-mercaptopurine to reduce clinical signs effectively in a severely unresponsive patient.

Less toxic agents, such as melphalan (Alkeran) and chlorambucil (Leukeran), have been used with variable success in patients that failed to respond to any other form of treatment. When one uses these drugs, the patient must be monitored weekly, to be sure that the leukocyte and thrombocyte counts, as well as the blood urea nitrogen, remain within normal limits.

Topical Preparations

In addition to topical steroids, a variety of topical preparations are often soothing and help to reduce irritation. They include such preparations as calamine lotion, Caladryl (combined calamine and diphenhydramine), colloidal sulfur lotion, Solarcaine (benzocaine and triclosan) and Unguentine (benzocaine) sprays and creams, sodium bicarbonate slurry or paste, and vinegar. As mentioned before, one must keep the dog occupied for 15 to 20 minutes after application of topical agents, to give the medication a chance to be absorbed before it is licked off. One must be particularly careful in selecting topical agents for cats because of their propensity to lick and groom, as well as their increased susceptibility to many therapeutic agents.

Aloe vera is an interesting botanical agent that has begun to receive serious attention during the past 10 years as an anti-inflammatory agent. Although aloe vera is not new—medical claims have been made for it for centuries—prior claims have been considered anecdotal, so only recent reports are considered to have merit. Its principal action seems to be its ability to block the production (or action) of prostaglandin and thromboxane, thereby reducing pain, inflammation, and itching. Laboratory studies also suggest that aloe vera may have some degree of antifungal and antibacterial activity.

REFERENCE

1. Soave, O., and Fuenzalida, E.: Effect of cortisone on antibody level of mice given rabies antigen three months earlier. Am. J. Vet. Res., *30*:643, 1969.

13 || *Food Allergy*

Food allergy fills a unique and curious niche in veterinary practice. It can be at once exasperating, exhilarating, confusing, obscure, frustrating, and satisfying, depending on how quickly the diagnosis is made and how stubbornly the patient responds. Yet once the clinician has become attuned to the problem, food allergy can also be among the simplest of allergic diseases to diagnose and manage.

The following case history illustrates just how frustrating the diagnosis and management of food allergy can sometimes be. A young, mixed-breed female dog was referred to me with a severe, nonseasonal pruritus that had begun when she was about 7 months old. Her history and clinical signs were consistent with a probable food allergy, and in fact, she responded well to food evaluation, consisting of an initial trial with cottage cheese, to which were added vegetables and cooked eggs at 5-day intervals. The pruritus had almost completely disappeared, when she suddenly began to regress. After a long and nonproductive discussion, the client suddenly asked whether changing the brand of cottage cheese could possibly make a difference. The client then explained that, initially, she had been using an expensive premium brand (A), but had decided to change to a less expensive chain-store brand (C) a few days before the dog's condition worsened.

Following a return to the initial brand of cottage cheese, the dog improved rapidly. When switched back to the chain-store brand, she again became much worse. When a third brand (B) of cottage cheese was tried, the dog developed a pruritus intermediate in intensity between that seen with brands A and C. This effect was reproducible for over 6 months, until the challenge was discontinued. Replies to my inquiries to the 3 dairy companies indicated that all three brands were apparently processed in the same way. One can only speculate on the reason, but the difference was probably in the milk supply and may have been a result of differences in pasture, fodder, or unknown factors.

Considering that food allergy is now the "darling" of the veterinary meeting circuit, with hardly a major program failing to devote at least one paper to its diagnosis and management, it is difficult to realize that until about 10 years ago, food allergy was among the most overlooked diagnoses in clinical medicine. Both its incidence and significance were grossly understated, and it was generally considered diagnostically unimportant.

HISTORICAL BACKGROUND

This situation is strange because, historically, food allergy is the oldest recognized form of allergy in animals. Veterinarians today often think that allergy, and particularly food allergy, is a recently discovered phenomenon. Yet when one searches the literature, we find case reports of animal food allergy in both the human and veterinary medical journals as early as 1920. The reason may, in part, be a loss in continuity caused by World War II. In spite of a rising interest in food allergy throughout the 1920s and 1930s, with even a faint spark of interest in the possibility of inhalant allergy, the war caused a massive change in emphasis in both human and veterinary medicine. By the time the war ended, we had entered the antibiotic age, followed by the corticosteroid, enzyme, and other "medical-miracle" eras. Older literature was often forgotten, and the new age of miracle drugs and miracle surgeries made practice more exciting than it had ever been before. There was just no time left for delving into food histories and performing other "archaic" procedures, such as talking to the client.

Some of the early cases were studied by physicians interested in comparative medicine who were intrigued by the close similarity between the clinical picture in "lower" animals and in man. In fact, much of what we now consider to be the pathogenesis of food allergy in animals has been extrapolated from human research because, except for the work done by Walton and Parrish, and perhaps a few others, no real scientific studies of this important problem have been conducted.[1–3]

The earliest confirmed case report of food allergy in animals appeared in 1920 and involved two sibling puppies that developed urticaria shortly after eating a meal of milk-based oyster stew. The puppies initially had pea-sized pruritic wheals that gradually enlarged and coalesced. Pruritus became intense, with vomiting and fever developing shortly thereafter. This report represents not only the first recorded case of food allergy in animals, but also the first familial or genetically associated case.

At about the same time, a report appeared in the *American Medical Journal,* the forerunner of *JAMA,* of an orphaned baby walrus that developed a severe and intractable hemorrhagic enteritis while being fed a cow's-milk formula. The disorder was diagnosed as cow's-milk allergy by the attending physician, and a change in diet resulted in a complete and permanent cure. Although this case was reported as allergy, one must wonder in retrospect whether this was a true allergy or an intolerance to lactase, lactalbumin, or some other component of milk.

The next published report came in 1922, when Phillips, also a physician, described two unrelated dogs with angioedema due to food sensitivity. The first was a 5-month-old English bulldog that began vomiting and developed angioedema, intense pruritus, and a profuse and, at times, bloody diarrhea after eating ham. When the dog was scratch tested 1 year later, he still showed a strong positive reaction to pork. The second case involved a cocker spaniel that had repeated attacks of angioedema that appeared suddenly as single wheals, often as large as half an orange, without other clinical signs. These attacks always followed the dog's being fed canned or fresh fish.

Regular reports continued to appear in the literature. By then, a few investigators were beginning to consider eczema a manifestation of food allergy, estimated to affect at least 15% of the canine population. Diagnostic skin testing for foods was recommended, but opinions varied on their reliability without a thorough dietary history. Among the common food allergens reported on the basis of both skin testing and history were salmon, cornmeal, wheat flour, potatoes, rice, pork, and eggs. In one study, 5 dogs with clinical signs were tested and found positive to a variety of food extracts. When these animals were subjected to provocative feeding tests, however, only 3 of the 5 dogs developed either skin or gastrointestinal signs. The investigator finally concluded that diet testing was the only reliable test procedure for food allergy.[4] If skin tests were to be given, however, he recommended that only the intradermal test be used because, in spite of its deficiencies, the other tests were too unreliable.

A comprehensive study was published in 1934 that reviewed and evaluated what was known about food allergy at that time.[5] A total of 76 dogs, 60 with normal skin and 16 with eczema or furunculosis, were skin tested with a variety of food antigens. Nineteen of the normal dogs (33%) and 9 of the affected dogs (56%) showed positive skin-test reactions. The principal positive reactions were obtained with salmon, wheat, alfalfa, and rice. Prousnitz-Kustner (P-K) tests were tried with serum from 8 of the dogs that reacted, and most showed antibody responses. Provocative feeding trials on dogs with both normal skin and positive test reactions failed to elicit a response. The study's conclusion was that skin tests were of limited value unless substantiated by feeding trials.

Other reports continued to appear sporadically during this period, but one additional study is worth mentioning. The author of this report described eight cases of food allergy resulting in either urticaria or hemorrhagic enteritis.[6] In the three dogs with urticaria, two were allergic to eggs and one to kibbled dog food. In the five dogs with hemorrhagic enteritis, three were allergic to horsemeat and one to kibble; one dog died before the allergen could be determined. One dog also had eczema, which cleared following dietary therapy.

During this period, cats were singularly absent from any literature reports, probably an indication of the low esteem in which the cat was held by many veterinarians at that time. This prior prejudice is especially ironic because cats represent a substantial number of the food allergy cases seen in veterinary allergists' offices.

Not until the work of Walton was published did well-documented cases of food allergy in cats become available. His reports on the pathologic changes in the gastrointestinal tract in food-induced enteric allergy are classics.

Lest one think that food allergy is limited to dogs and cats among domestic animal species, cattle can be allergic to ingested foods, such as milk, concentrates, hay, grain, silage, pasture, and potato leaves. Clinically, cattle have urticaria, slight respiratory distress, and gastrointestinal signs. Some reports also describe allergic reactions to foods in horses.

INCIDENCE

Overall Incidence

Reliable figures are not available for the overall incidence of food-induced allergies in animals because most published reports deal with individual case histories and diagnostic procedures, rather than incidence. Furthermore, food allergy is often misdiagnosed and the cause variously ascribed to other factors. Until recently, most veterinarians did not think of food as a cause of allergy, so it was often overlooked as a diagnosis. Therefore, published figures are unreliable, at best.

In 1967, Walton reported on food-allergic skin disease in 82 dogs and 16 cats presented at the dermatology clinic of the University of Liverpool, England.[1] Based on these figures, he estimated that about 1% of skin cases seen in a general veterinary practice are due to food. In my opinion, this figure does not represent the true incidence of food allergy because it does not include nondermatologic

cases involving the gastrointestinal tract and other organ systems. This percentage also overlooks the subclinical food allergies that do not become manifest unless coupled with a subclinical inhalant allergy.

Finally, Walton's incidence figures are also skewed by showing them as a percentage of all dermatologic cases entering the clinic, rather than as representative only of nonseasonal allergy. To illustrate the point, many years ago I did a retrospective review of 82 consecutive cases of nonseasonal allergic dermatitis and found that food was wholly or partially responsible for the clinical signs in 62% of the cases reviewed. Of the total group, in 23% signs cleared completely following dietary therapy, and 39% of these patients showed partial improvement. These figures closely correlated with those derived by another investigator several years later. It is important to remember that many allergic dogs have sensitivities to both food and inhalants, and these dogs must be included in both categories when calculating incidence.

Breed Incidence

No definitive studies of breed incidence have been conducted, and all the common breeds in my practice area seem to be represented (Table 13–1). In terms of overall al-

Table 13–1.   Breeds Represented in 82 Cases of Nonseasonal Allergic Dermatitis

Mixed breed	17
German shepherd	24
Poodle	7
Golden retriever	4
Collie	4
Wirehaired fox terrier	4
Springer spaniel	3
Airedale	2
Japanese spaniel	1
Miniature schnauzer	1
Shih-Tzu	1
Dalmatian	1
Weimaraner	1
Bouvier	1
Welsh terrier	1
Irish setter	1
West Highland white terrier	1
Doberman pinscher	1
Dachshund	1
Fox terrier	1
Cocker spaniel	1
Scottish terrier	1
Cats	3
(1 Siamese, 2 domestic short-haired)	

lergy, however, German shepherds and golden retrievers seemed to be overrepresented in the review cited previously, even given the popularity of German shepherds at the time. The number of golden retrievers is particularly interesting. In spite of the low number reported, these figures were gathered before the golden retriever achieved its current popularity as a family pet. Therefore, they actually represented a higher percentage of golden retrievers than was generally seen in an average practice at that time.

No doubt these breed incidence figures are different from those reported by other investigators, partly because of the breed popularity index in any given practice area. More important, however, Table 13–1 represents a study of **nonseasonally allergic dogs and cats only,** and therefore the percentage of cases is much higher than would be found in a random population or in seasonally allergic animals.

ETIOLOGY

Food antigens, like other allergens, are usually protein molecules with a molecular weight of 10,000 daltons or more; however, reactions have also been caused by glycoproteins, lipoproteins, lipopolysaccharides, carbohydrates, and some small molecules acting as haptens. Small, haptenic molecules are not always obvious, and sensitivity reactions in man have been reported from hidden, unlabeled dyes and other agents in foods, beverages, and drugs. Agents known or suspected of causing allergic or other adverse reactions include artificial colors, flavors, and preservatives. Allergic reactions may be caused by the compound itself, if it is of proper size and configuration to constitute an antigen or, in the case of a hapten, by the complete antigen formed after it combines with a carrier protein.

One can only speculate whether this factor may be responsible for the reactions frequently seen when animals eat pet foods because formulations are trade secrets. It is certainly not uncommon to find some animals that react to canned beef, lamb, or other pet foods that do not react to the same food when fed fresh. This difference, of course, also may reflect molecular changes caused by processing.

Unsuspected drugs in foods also can cause reactions. Walton and Parish published an interesting report of a farm cat that developed severe intestinal allergic reactions to milk containing penicillin residues.[2] Uncontaminated milk was tolerated without incident, but when the cat was challenged later with oral penicillin, clinical signs again returned.

Some foods, such as egg white, in addition to their allergenic potential, are also nonspecific histamine releasers. Although this problem is uncommon, such foods may cause nonspecific histamine release from mast cells, mimicking an allergic reaction, without the actual presence of an antigen/antibody reaction.

Opinions differ on which foods are most allergenic based on geographic area, culinary cultural habits, and food fads. Therefore, no two lists are identical, even from the same locale. Obviously, rarely fed foods are not significant on any list, and highly allergenic foods appear frequently. The most extensive study, again, is that of Walton (Table 13–2), as described previously.[1]

In my experience, the greatest number of food-associated problems in dogs and cats follow the feeding of commercial dog and cat foods, biscuits, and dog treats. This situation probably reflects the feeding habits of pet owners in the United States, where prepared canned and dry foods constitute the principal diet of most pets. In addition, unknown additives and changes in the food because of processing temperatures and pressures may also influence the development of these reactions.

Factors contributing to the onset and development of clinical signs associated with food allergy include "loading factors" and the "allergic threshold." Loading factors are additional allergens or other factors that, when combined with a low-grade allergy, initiate an allergic reaction. For example, although food-allergic patients usually have clinical problems throughout the year, a patient may have a subclinical allergy to a food, as well as a subclinical allergy to an inhalant. Exposure to only one class of allergens may not elicit a reaction, but when that allergen

Table 13–2. Incidence of Allergenic Foods in Study by Walton

DOG		CAT	
Food	Number	Food	Number
Milk	23	Milk	7
Canned dog food	17	Cooked beef	4
Wheat	10	Raw beef	1
Raw beef	9	Chicken	1
Cooked beef	4	Penicillin	1
Dog biscuits	4	Rabbit	1
Eggs	3	Cat food	1

(From Walton, G.S.: Skin responses in the dog and cat to ingested allergens: observations on 100 confirmed cases. Vet. Rec., *81*:709, 1967.)

is combined with another type of allergen, the reaction may be exponential, rather than additive, with a resultant severe clinical problem. In such a case, the problem would occur seasonally, but would still be partially caused by a food allergy.

The allergic threshold, on the other hand, is the degree of exposure required to trigger an attack. In this situation, individuals may develop a sensitivity to a specific food, yet tolerate it when fed that food either infrequently or in small amounts.

Finally, allergic reactions may follow the ingestion of some specific food as a result of sensitivity to something used in preparation, rather than to the food itself. In such cases, the food becomes the carrier of the actual allergenic substance. For example, bread that has been leavened by yeast, or cheese that develops its particular characteristics because of mold, may cause reactions in individuals with fungal inhalant sensitivities. Milk from cows recently treated with penicillin may contain enough penicillin residue to cause a reaction in penicillin-sensitive individuals.

SENSITIVITY VERSUS INTOLERANCE AND PSEUDOALLERGY

The general tendency is to classify all reactions following the ingestion of food or other substances as allergic, regardless of the true underlying cause. In fact, for a reaction to be truly allergic, antibodies must be involved and the reaction must be immediate, at least in a kinetic sense. Although immunoglobulins E (IgE)-mediated Type I reactions are involved in most food-associated allergic diseases, numerous studies have shown that these allergies may also be due to Type III and Type IV reactions, and food allergy may be associated with IgA, IgG, IgM, complement, or sensitized lymphocytes. Type II reactions have been reported, but the evidence for these reactions is questionable. Therefore, although technically one should only refer to Type I reactions as food **allergy,** in actual practice, food allergy and food hypersensitivity are used interchangeably, as long as an immune reaction is involved.

To compound the problem further, food allergy must be distinguished from intolerance and, possibly, from pseudoallergy (false food allergy).

False Food Allergy

Pseudoallergy has been recognized and described in man, but no studies have yet been done to prove its occurrence in animals. Cases have been seen in dogs with clinical signs similar to those seen in people, however, so we have good reason to suspect that it probably also occurs in dogs. Pseudoallergy is generally caused by certain foods and chemicals, particularly food additives, colors, and preservatives, that either contain high concentrations of biogenic amines, such as histamine or tyramine, or are capable of liberating inflammatory mediators from the mast cell. These substances do not act as allergens, yet produce clinical problems closely resembling food allergy. Unlike allergy, in which minute quantities are often enough to initiate an immune response, large amounts of food are generally required to cause a false-allergy reaction. The principal foods of interest to veterinarians include egg white, shellfish, pork, canned and frozen fish, fermented foods, such as cheeses, and chocolate. These biogenic amines can also be produced locally in the intestinal tract by bacterial fermentation, particularly of carbohydrates.

Although many clinical signs are associated with false allergy in man, those of interest to veterinarians are limited to urticaria, angioedema, and diarrhea. For example, a young adult male boxer was once brought in with diarrhea and severe angioedema of the entire body after eating part of a bucket of chum (a mixture of ground fish and shellfish used as bait while trolling for deep-sea fish). He had had no problem with fish in the past and did not react to a challenge with small quantities at a later date. This disorder was classified as a food-allergy reaction at the time, but in retrospect, it may well have represented a false-allergy reaction. Given that dyes and other artificial colors have been incriminated in false-food-allergy reactions in man, one must wonder whether some of the "food allergy" reactions associated with the deeply red-colored soft-moist foods fed to animals may represent false allergy. Finally, some of the skin and gastrointestinal problems occasionally seen following ingestion of dry dog foods may possibly be due to bacterial fermentation of carbohydrates with release of biogenic amines and may represent false allergy rather than true food allergy. This is not to say that these conditions are not caused by food allergy, but that other possibilities must also be considered and explored.

Even though pseudofood allergy has received no attention in veterinary medicine, one should consider it in any patient with urticaria of sudden onset that is not recurrent, for which an allergic or other cause, e.g., bee stings or other insect venoms, cannot be found. Diagnostic criteria established for man are based on allergy skin tests for known food allergens, maintenance of a diet diary, and provocation testing with either the biogenic amines or suspected foods. These substances must be given in small amounts, and if a reaction occurs, it is probably allergy. When large amounts are required to induce a reaction, it is probably false allergy.

Intolerance

Intolerance, on the other hand, is much more difficult to define or to categorize than pseudoallergy and can be due to a variety of pharmacologic, toxic, idiosyncratic, and physiologic defects or changes. These changes include gastric achlorhydria, pancreatic enzyme deficiencies, changes in gastrointestinal motility and other mechanical factors, reduced bile secretions, and any other factor interfering with normal breakdown and absorption of foods. Clinical signs are generally related to the gastrointestinal tract, rather than to the skin or other organ systems.

PATHOGENESIS OF FOOD ALLERGY

The chain of events ultimately leading to the production of clinical signs is incompletely understood. In human medicine, food allergy is of great interest to allergists, immunologists, and gastroenterologists, so ongoing research to elucidate its mechanisms is extensive. Although much of the following has been extrapolated from the human literature, most of the basic principles probably apply to animals, as well. Even if they are not directly applicable, one should still understand what is known about food allergy in people, to better understand food allergy in general.

Antibodies

IgE is probably the principal antibody in food allergy, although other classes of antibodies are also involved. Regardless of whether the reaction is Type I, III, or IV, it is still an immune reaction. That inflammatory mediators released by intestinal mucosal mast cells are involved is amply demonstrated experimentally by the protective effect of cromolyn sodium when that agent is given orally before challenging the patient with known food allergens. In addition, prostaglandin-synthetase inhibitors have been of value in treating ulcerative colitis and diarrhea in man, and another study showed that prophylactic doses of aspirin, indomethacin, and ibuprofen prevented symptoms of food sensitivity in five of six patients. Serotonin, released by the chromaffin cells of the lamina propria, may also be a mediator in the induction of food allergy.

Mucosal Immune System

The mucosal immune system, separate and distinct from the systemic immune system, apparently plays some role in the protection against food allergy. This is a highly complex system, consisting of macrophages, mast cells, natural killer cells, intraepithelial lymphocytes, and B and T lymphocytes residing in the lamina propria. The function of the mucosal immune system is to protect the body against invasion through mucosal surfaces. The specific sequence of events leading to protection—or lack thereof—in food allergy is poorly understood, although it is generally accepted that secretory IgA plays a protective role.

Factors in the Onset of Reaction

The reaction may occur immediately after eating, or it may occur 1 to many hours after ingestion. The onset of the reaction is influenced by many factors, such as

1. Whether the allergen is soluble or insoluble
2. Emptying time of the stomach
3. Intestinal motility
4. Presence of intestinal inflammatory lesions
5. Whether the reaction is due to a whole food molecule or one changed by acid hydrolysis or digestion

Most nutrients enter the circulation through the normal processes of digestion and absorption. Insoluble food particles and other large molecules, however, may enter the circulation through the lymphatic system by direct passage through the intestinal wall by a process called "persorption." In persorption, particles are forced between the cells of the intestinal wall with the help of intestinal muscular movements. These powerful forces cause openings in the intercellular spaces large enough to allow large particles to pass directly into the lymphatic vessels and eventually to enter the circulation through the thoracic duct.

As early as 1913, researchers demonstrated that whole protein molecules could be absorbed directly into the circulation without digestive breakdown.[7] In this study, the stomach of a dog was isolated, and milk was placed directly into its lumen. Blood drawn 2 hours later had enough milk protein to cause anaphylaxis in sensitized guinea pigs. Whole protein absorption was further demonstrated in 1926, when horse serum injected into a ligated loop of a guinea pig's small intestine was absorbed intact.[7]

Other factors are also apparently important in the absorption of whole food particles or the increased absorption of potentially allergenic particles. Age is important in man; the immature gut of infants absorbs many more antigenic particles than the more mature gut of the adult. This difference is due, in part, to the lag time between birth and the development of a protective layer of glycocalyx and secretory IgA. The glycocalyx is a gluey glycoprotein secretion coating the gastrointestinal epithelial cells, thus acting as a mechanical barrier to the random absorption of large molecules, while secretory IgA lines the intestinal tract and traps infectious and other antigenic particles.

Protective Antibody

Strong evidence supports the protective role of IgA in food allergy. A study in man, for example, has shown that children with lower-than-normal IgA levels are much more likely to develop precipitating antibody to cow's milk than normal children. Other excellent studies suggest that withholding foods likely to cause food allergy until at least 9 months of age significantly reduces the incidence of food allergy in children from families with a medical history predictive of a much higher incidence. By 9 months of age, secretory IgA begins to coat the intestinal tract, and as the child matures, the concentration of IgA increases and becomes more protective, finally reaching adult levels at about 4 years. Physically, this substance is sticky, and when present in adequate quantities, virtually lines the intestinal tract. Therefore, withholding allergenic foods until adequate IgA is present in the gut appears to be helpful in delaying, or preventing, the onset of food allergy.

These same factors are probably also involved in the development of food allergy in the dog and cat. Puppies and kittens are weaned much younger than they would be in nature, often by 4 to 5 weeks, and are placed on some type of commercially prepared pet food, milk, or other solid food. Because the gut is still immature at this time, potentially allergenic particles are absorbed in high concentration and predispose the pet to food allergy. In all probability, this is why so many animals exhibit their first clinical signs when they are between 6 and 9 months old.

Nonimmune Factors

Villous erosions, ulcerations, and other inflammatory intestinal lesions caused by toxic or infectious processes increase the diffusion of large food particles across the damaged mucosa and into the circulation and thereby increase the probability of food allergy. Pancreatic deficiency also contributes to the development of food hypersensitivity because of the lack of sufficient breakdown of macromolecules and enhanced absorption of these large particles.

Macrophages, in concert with IgA and lysosomes, help to maintain the integrity of the intestinal barrier. Therefore, any alteration of the homeostasis of the gastrointestinal host defenses can increase the absorption of large molecules and the consequent possibility of the induction of an allergic response.

The failure to release lysosomal enzymes from the digestive vacuoles of intestinal absorptive cells may be another contributing factor. At the cellular level, these enzymes are involved in the final breakdown of most ingested material. Therefore, any interference with intracellular release can also enhance absorption of large molecules. Because corticosteroids are believed to stabilize the lysosomal membrane, one must also consider the possibility that corticosteroid use may interfere with lysosomal enzyme digestive function and cause enhanced transmucosal transport of antigens.

Even the developing fetus is not entirely spared from the induction of food allergy. A report on intrauterine sensitization to egg white in newborn infants suggests that prenatal sensitivity can also occur. The investigators demonstrated IgE antibody production prenatally, with resulting atopic dermatitis involving the cheeks, chin, thigh, and abdomen of newborn infants. How similar this is to the clinical signs of food allergy commonly seen in cats.

Pathologic Changes

Except for the work of Walton, little has appeared in the veterinary literature describing pathologic changes associated with the allergic response. In the excellent case report cited previously, in which Walton confirmed a case of milk allergy in a cat by both skin tests and provocative challenge, he also found high titers of agglutinating antibodies to milk proteins, particularly lactalbumin, and especially after periods of milk feeding. In addition, 1 of 8 cats on which passive cutaneous anaphylaxis (PCA) tests were performed exhibited positive reactions.

In the foregoing study, intestinal biopsy sections taken both before and after provocative challenge showed significant changes in the allergically reacting gut. The number of plasma cells in the lamina propria was markedly increased, with degeneration of some of the tips of the villi and mild hemorrhage into the lumen. These animals also had edema of the submucosa and clots containing shreds of epithelium. Pathologic changes appeared to be more severe in the colon than in the ileum and jejunum. These findings are similar to those seen on biopsy in man.

CLINICAL SIGNS

Reactions may be immediate or delayed, in a temporal rather than an immunologic sense. Depending on the rapidity of food absorption into the lymphatic and general circulation, a food-allergic reaction can occur within minutes or hours. This variation can be due to a number of factors, including solubility of the particular food, rate of intestinal motility, and level of digestion to which the patient is allergic; for example, is the allergy caused by the whole food molecule or one of the chain of digestive breakdown products?

Skin

The most common dermal sign of food allergy is pruritus, which generally is intense and may or may not be accompanied by skin

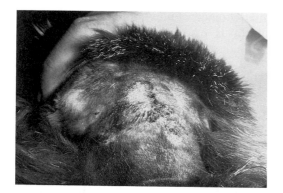

Fig. 13–1.   Severe allergic dermatitis with alopecia and ulceration.

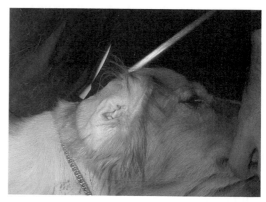

Fig. 13–3.   Allergic otitis with pinnal erythema and edema in a golden retriever.

lesions. In fact, food allergy should be at the top of any differential diagnosis list for a patient presented with pruritus but with no obviously observable gross lesions.

Clinically, skin lesions range from no grossly visible lesions to severe, ulcerative dermatitis. The early signs may be nothing more than a dry, thin, lifeless coat with a light, flaking scale or dander. As lesions progress, one sees erythema, scaling, crusts, excoriations, hyperkeratosis, seborrhea, alopecia, pigmentation, and ulceration (Fig. 13–1). Urticaria and angioedema also are seen occasionally (Fig. 13–2), as is otitis with pinnal erythema and edema (Fig. 13–3). In the dog, lesions can appear anywhere on the body, although urticaria and angioedema occur most commonly on the face and trunk. Except for urticaria and angioedema, which usually are not seen in inhalant allergy, little distinguishes the signs of food allergy from those of other forms of allergic disease in the dog.

The cat, on the other hand, is more likely to have lesions around the face, head, neck, and shoulders, and these lesions are commonly much more ulcerative or deeply erosive than in the dog (Fig. 13–4). Because ulceration is the most frequent manifestation of food allergy in this species, it must be differentiated from other ulcerative dermatitides, such as rodent ulcer, "eosinophilic granuloma complex," dermal lymphosarcoma, and autoimmune diseases. Another common manifestation of food allergy in cats is so-called miliary dermatitis (Fig. 13–5),

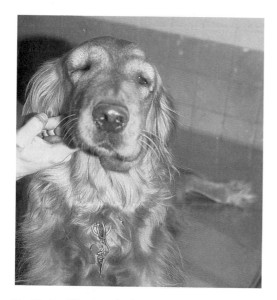

Fig. 13–2.   Allergic urticaria and angioedema in a golden retriever.

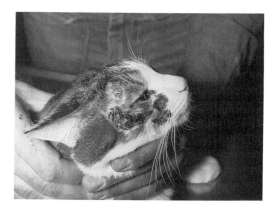

Fig. 13–4.   Ulcerative allergic dermatitis in a cat.

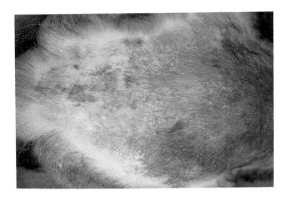

Fig. 13–5. Allergic miliary dermatitis in a cat.

although this disorder can be a manifestation of other diseases, as well.

Why the most common clinical signs of food allergy should involve the skin, rather than the gut or other organs, is difficult to explain. Certainly, more than adequate numbers of mast cells are present in the lamina propria of the gut, pulmonary tissue, and other organs. Moreover, one would assume that because food is in intimate contact with the gut and all its associated immune organ structures, the gastrointestinal tract should logically be the most common system involved in food allergy. Therefore, except for the rather weak explanation that "the skin is the primary target organ" for allergy in the dog, and perhaps in the cat, we will have to await proper studies for a better explanation.

This aspect of food allergy has not been elucidated in man, either. Gell and Coombs have suggested that food allergy be divided into two broad groups: (1) "gastrointestinal allergy," for reactions such as vomiting, diarrhea, and colic occurring within the gastrointestinal tract; and (2) "alimentary allergy," for all those outside the gastrointestinal tract, such as asthma, dermatitis, and migraine.

In another attempt to make the terminology more precise, two broad general areas have been defined and classified: food allergy and gastrointestinal allergy. These areas are not considered the same; food allergy affects all organ systems, and gastrointestinal allergy affects only the gastrointestinal tract. In addition, gastrointestinal reactions are occasionally caused by allergens other than food, such as drugs, chemicals, inhalants, or in-

jected agents. Furthermore, although the concept is well established, descriptive differences do exist among some authorities.[8]

The diverse clinical syndromes and subclasses of food-associated allergy described in man are not universally accepted. Furthermore, only in recent years has food allergy begun to receive more attention in veterinary medicine, and little has yet been done to elucidate its pathobiologic mechanisms and many possible associated syndromes. Therefore, veterinarians should overlook these divisions for now and just refer to food allergy or food hypersensitivity, regardless of where the reaction occurs.

Gastrointestinal Tract

Intestinal signs may be acute or chronic and may vary from mild to severe. As the condition continues or becomes progressive, one sees weight loss, unthriftiness, and general debility.

In the acute form, onset is sudden with a severe, usually profuse and watery, diarrhea. Shortly thereafter, the stools may become bloody, and free blood may even be present in the intestinal lumen. Strands and clumps of mucus are present, and the diarrhea has a foul stench reminiscent of an open sewer. In spite of the acute signs, the dog does not generally seem to be in any great distress and is usually alert, active, and even playful. This syndrome is so consistent as to warrant a presumptive diagnosis of food allergy until proved otherwise.

This specificity does not mean that one can forego a proper diagnostic workup. Because medicine has no absolutes, a complete history must still be taken, and a complete general physical and abdominal examination, including radiographs if necessary, must be made.

Treatment consists of the parenteral administration of 5 mg or more of prednisolone, depending on the size of the dog, or other suitable corticosteroid and 50 to 100 mg diphenhydramine. Response to treatment is rapid, and stools usually return to normal in about 6 hours.

The chronic form is much more variable, with clinical signs ranging from nothing more than eructation or flatulence, to occasional or daily vomiting, mucoid stools, intestinal rumbling, soft stools, and occasional or cyclic diarrhea. Stools are usually soft or mushy, rather than watery, and are often coated with mucus. Frank blood is rare. The skin may be dry and scaly, and the hair coat harsh, dry, and rough, epilating easily.

In a study of 60 allergic people with colic, diarrhea, and vomiting, eosinophilia persisted in the stool mucus until the offending foods were removed from the diet. This situation has not yet been studied in veterinary medicine, but, checking the stool for eosinophilia is certainly worth investigating as another possible diagnostic tool.

Other Organ Systems

Food-allergic reactions in other organ systems have not been as well documented in animals as in man, but more than enough suggestive clinical evidence supports their existence.

Urinary Tract

Recurrent cystitis, including hemorrhagic cystitis, has been seen, particularly in cats. In a recent clinical study of feline cystitis by Thorsen in California, the cats in the series underwent complete remission as a result of his altering their diets.[9] Cases were evaluated by skin tests, bladder biopsy, and food trial. When the suspect foods were withdrawn, improvement was quickly apparent. When the offending foods were reintroduced, clinical signs returned. Dr. Thorsen concluded that magnesium oxide is not the principal agent responsible for feline urinary syndrome. Consequently, recurrent cystitis should be considered a food allergy until proved otherwise, with proper dietary control as the key to management.

Evidence also suggests that some cases of immune-mediated glomerulonephritis in man may be the result of the complexing of antibody wih food antigens. Some cases of enuresis in children are also thought to be due to food allergy, although agreement is not universal on this issue.

Respiratory Tract

Asthma and other respiratory problems, though not common, may also be due to foods. Although occasionally seen in dogs, asthma is much more likely in cats.

Nervous System

The neurologic system may be affected in several ways. I have seen food-associated epileptiform seizures, and so have other veterinarians treating food allergy. Collins described several dogs that he had treated with convulsive disorders that became clinically normal following dietary adjustment.[10] The effect was reproducible because seizures returned when the offending foods were again fed.

Behavioral changes seen in dogs with food allergies are suggestive of the work of the late Dr. Feingold of San Francisco, who described a series of hyperkinetic children who had difficulty resting and concentrating, were constantly active, and did poorly in school. Dr. Feingold ascribed many of their problems to food additives, such as artificial colors, flavors, and preservatives. When the children's diets were changed, many experienced a change in attitude and behavior; they became much easier to live with, and their ability to learn improved significantly.

In man, other reported central nervous system reactions include behavior problems, hyperirritability, insomnia, and drowsiness. In addition, an estimated 20% of milk-sensitive infants have been reported to have behavioral changes.

Similar changes also occur in dogs. Following a fast diet change, many owners report a distinct improvement in personality and behavior. Common comments include: "he seems so much more relaxed and sleeps better at night," "he's doing things he hasn't done for years—he's become playful again and seems so much more interested in what's going on around him."

Even changes in temperament are noted. A classic example involves a dog I treated a few years ago that had a food-allergic dermatitis and one of the worst temperaments I had ever seen. He was snappy, irritable, and extremely difficult to handle. Not only was he untrustworthy around strangers, he even bit his own family on occasion.

During the initial diagnostic fasting period described later in this chapter, all toys were removed, along with the food. This included such things as rubber and plastic balls, stuffed toys, rawhide, and chewsticks. When the dog had been without food for 3 days, the owner called to report that the dermatitis had improved markedly, and the dog had also had a remarkable improvement in disposition. Although the dog had not actually become trustworthy, he was not as easily provoked to bite the family as before.

After several weeks, he was again allowed to play with his favorite ball, and about 8 hours later, his temperament became much worse. He became more aggressive and much more difficult to handle. The ball was taken away, and within 24 hours, the dog's temperament had again improved. This process was repeated several times, with the same results. Because of the length of time it took for changes both to develop and to abate after introduction and removal of the ball, we reasonably ruled out possessiveness and assumed he was reacting to the curing agents or some other chemical within the ball. It is difficult to know just which chemical(s) he was reacting to because it could have been the latex itself or one of the many curing agents, binders, or dyes.

In another case involving an aggressive, irritable, unpredictable Lhasa apso, with food sensitivity as a major part of its allergic problem, the owner reported a dramatic improvement in behavior following dietary adjustment and elimination of the foods to which it was allergic.

Cardiovascular System

Cardiovascular signs have not been recognized in the dog or cat, but fascinating work in human medicine should alert us to this possibility. In one study of the effects of foods, environment, and ingestant contaminants, 1 patient developed reproducible hypotension, shock, and fibrillation following ingestion of milk and eggs. In addition, 10 of 12 patients placed and studied in environmentally controlled rooms showed clear-cut cardiac reactions to food or contaminants in the drinking water when the patients were given a provocative diet. No patient had isolated heart involvement without symptoms relating to other smooth muscle organs.

Symptoms ranged from minimal in some patients to severe and seemingly life-threatening in others.

Finally, evidence indicates that some cases of myocardial infarction may be due to allergy, in which coronary artery spasm occurs without atherosclerosis. When foods have been implicated, a correlation has been noted between probable cause of mortality and serum antibodies to cow's-milk protein and egg white. In this study, samples taken soon after myocardial infarction were predictive of mortality during the following 6 months when antibody to these 2 food proteins was present.

DIAGNOSIS

The diagnosis of food allergy can sometimes be challenging, summoning all the veterinarian's diagnostic skills. A proper evaluation is contingent upon

1. History
2. Physical examination
3. Appropriate laboratory tests
4. Other diagnostic tests and provocative challenge

History

At the risk of beating an old maxim to death, in food allergy, as in any other area of diagnosis, no substitute exists for a thorough medical history. This step is the first and most important in the diagnostic workup. As noted in Chapter 4, one should develop and use a standard history form, so important information is not overlooked. Obtain a general pattern of daily feeding habits, and note whether any correlation exists between the time and type of feeding and the onset of clinical signs. The owner should be particularly observant about the possible presence of gastrointestinal changes. Try to determine whether there is a difference in the ability of the patient to tolerate specific foods when fed cooked than when fed raw and whether the onset or remission of clinical signs can be related to changes in the feeding pattern.

Signs of food allergy frequently appear early in life and are generally nonseasonal, although seasonal variations may occur because of loading factors, such as the additive effects of multiple exposures to subclinical allergens, and allergic threshold, as discussed earlier in this chapter.

Studies in man have shown that food-associated seasonal problems can also develop when certain foods are eaten by some pollen-allergic patients. For example, apples may cause oral itching in patients with birch pollinosis, celery and spices can cause angioedema in patients allergic to mugwort, and various melons can cause oral itching in ragweed-allergic people. This is probably due to the presence of shared allergens in the food and the pollen and probably represents an inhalant allergy, rather than a true food allergy, even though a food is actually triggering the reaction. Finally, it is conceivable that a subclinical food allergy in the presence of a subclinical inhalant sensitivity can provoke a clinical response.

In general, then, once you have ruled out fleas, sarcoptes, and other ectoparasites, food allergy should head the list of suspected diagnoses in any dog or cat with a pruritic problem that begins before the animal is 1 year old, particularly if it starts between the ages of 6 and 9 months. Furthermore, all patients with nonseasonal pruritus or dermatitis must be evaluated for food allergy before skin tests for inhalant or environmental allergens are given. It would be a colossal waste of time and money to perform skin tests for inhalants and then put the patient through a course of immunotherapy, only to discover that the principal problem is food.

Inquire about gastrointestinal signs. Most clients bringing a patient in for the treatment of a skin problem do not associate vomiting or diarrhea with the skin disease and do not think of offering this information voluntarily. Yet if food allergy is the cause, the patient often has a pattern of burping, cyclic vomiting and diarrhea, or soft, mushy, or mucoid stools. If such information is to be obtained, one must question the client.

Physical Examination

Examining a patient with food allergy is not remarkably different from examining one with inhalant allergy, except in relation to intestinal signs. To help to identify obstructive lesions in a vomiting or diarrheic patient, one should palpate the abdomen carefully and use sedation, if necessary, for deep palpation. Rectal examinations should be done and rectal smears examined for motile larvae, protozoa, and bacteria.

Appropriate Laboratory Tests

Laboratory tests are basically the same as for inhalant allergy, with a few additions. Skin scrapings, of course, are mandatory in any skin disease. Complete blood and differential counts, serum chemistries, and urinalysis are always desirable and should be part of every initial examination. Bacterial and fungal cultures should be performed, if pyoderma is present or if the lesions resemble dermatophyte infection. Biopsies should be taken, especially of the deeply erosive lesions often seen in cats.

When animals are presented with gastrointestinal problems, diagnostic radiography may be necessary to rule out obstructions, ulcers, and other lesions. Fecal mucus smears should also be made and examined for free blood and eosinophils. Fecal examination must also be performed, not only for routine intestinal parasites, but also for protozoan infections and bacteria. Stool culture can be helpful in persistently abnormal stools.

Immune Assays

The principal diagnostic procedures are allergy skin tests and the various forms of elimination diets. To these procedures can be added the recently introduced in vitro immune assays, the radioallergosorbent test (RAST) and enzyme-linked immunosorbent assay (ELISA) tests.

RAST and ELISA cannot be recommended for the diagnosis of food allergy at this time because they are both relatively new techniques in veterinary medicine and still unproved in food allergy. One problem associated with these tests is that ELISA and RAST are tests for IgE and not all food allergy is IgE mediated, but may also be associated with IgG, IgM, complement, and possibly, activated lymphocytes. In addition, an individual can be allergic to either the raw or cooked form (or both) of a particular food, or the whole food or a digestive breakdown product, and antigenic cross-reactivity may not exist among the various physical and digestive breakdown products. Under these circumstances, which food, and in which form, would one test? Obviously, both false-positive and false-negative results are likely.

Skin Tests

Allergy skin testing is also controversial; proponents and opponents vigorously line up on both sides of the issue. Many physician allergists consider the test to be reliable, but usually after they have reasonably identified the offending food through both history and observation.

Many studies in dogs during the 1930s and 1940s proved allergy skin tests for foods to be unreliable; positive-reacting foods failed to cause clinical signs, whereas negative reactors often caused lesions to develop. Some of the poor results could have been due to both the standardization and quality of the test extracts available at that time. The results of more recent evaluations have not been appreciably better, however.

Several possible reasons exist for poor skin test results, among them those cited previously for immune assays, namely, type of antigen (raw or cooked and whole or digested) and class of immune reaction. In addition, some food extracts contain naturally occurring histamine, which can provoke a false-positive wheal. Histamine can also be formed and incorporated into the extract by bacterial action on histadine during processing.

Physical factors, such as whether the food is soluble or insoluble, can affect the reliability of food tests. Evidence suggests that insoluble substances, such as starch granules, muscle fibers, cell walls, and other insoluble cell particles, can be allergenic. Because an extract cannot be made from an insoluble substance, test solutions would not contain these allergens and would, therefore, be of little value in diagnosing food allergy caused by these substances.

Other reasons for the unreliability of skin test extracts include loss of antigenic components during extraction and processing procedures, primary irritant properties of some extracts producing false-positive reactions, and nonspecific histamine-releasing properties of some food extracts. Finally, some investigators believe that fresh, or fresh-frozen, extracts are far more reliable than commercial antigens for skin testing.

In an article I wrote on this topic several years ago,[12] I said that Lietze, in reviewing the literature, lists 10 contributing causes, several of which may be applicable to veterinary practice.[7] These are (1) dilution of antigen due to incomplete purification; (2) insoluble allergens from which antigen cannot be extracted; (3) allergens that form as a result of digestion; (4) certain antigens that require chemical reactions with reducing sugars to become allergens; (5) fruit extracts, which lose their antigenicity if more than 24 hours old; (6) allergens prepared by different manufacturers, which may differ widely in potency and may actually be inactive; (7) endogenous blocking antibodies that may be present; (8) some food allergens that may exist as haptens and not become allergenic until they combine with body protein; (9) binding of circulating antibody by large amounts of antigens present in the ingests; and (10) the situation in which only the target organ may be sensitive to the antigen. Thus, if the target organ is the intestinal tract, the skin may not react to tests.

Immediate and delayed-onset clinical reactions also seem to affect the reliability of skin tests. In one study, skin tests were frequently positive in immediate-onset reactions, but much less so in delayed-onset reactions. The authors concluded that immediate-onset reactions can usually be diagnosed from history alone, and therefore skin testing or other tests are rarely indicated.[11] Another study in man concluded that allergy to soluble food antigens could frequently be diagnosed by history and skin tests, whereas allergy to insoluble food antigens can be diagnosed only by elimination and trial diet.

Food Elimination

The most reliable tests, then, involve direct food trials in patients. These trials can be performed in two ways: (1) feeding a restricted diet, usually lamb and rice or chicken and rice, for 3 weeks; or (2) totally eliminating food for 3 days and then starting a trial diet.

Restricted Diet

Although it is more readily accepted by the client, the restricted diet has one major defect. If the patient is sensitive to the trial food, improvement is then impossible. I commonly see patients with a history of possible allergy that have been referred for evaluation, with the referring veterinarians saying "we know it's not food allergy. He's been on lamb and rice for 3 weeks and hasn't improved." When the animal is fasted and placed on a trial diet, however, the improvement is often rapid and dramatic. If the patient is allergic to lamb or rice, the trial diet will not have proved a thing.

Cooking and processing can also affect the allergenicity of a food. A patient fed a commercial lamb and rice diet, or lamb baby food, may not show improvement, only to improve when given fresh lamb.

Rice itself also is not innocuous and may be allergenic. In a recent study, rice was reported to be the fifth most allergenic food for children. No figures are available on the incidence of rice sensitivity in dogs and cats, but three of my canine patients in a 6-month period reacted unfavorably to rice.

Fast and Trial Diet

The diagnostic procedure of choice is often referred to as an elimination diet, but it differs from the procedure as described for man. In people, groups of foods are eliminated from the diet for a specified period of time while the patient is observed for signs of improvement. As the term is used here, it actually refers to a 3-day fast followed by specific food trials, a procedure I call the fast-and-trial diet.

The client is instructed to administer a mild saline cathartic, such as milk of magnesia or Epsom salts, to hasten the elimination of food residues from the intestinal tract. No food is fed for 3 days, and the client is instructed to give the patient only bottled spring water for drinking, to remove all toys, and not to feed snacks. It may seem strange to find it necessary to remind the client about snacks and tidbits, but many clients do not equate such things with food and feed them unless specifically instructed otherwise. The water source is changed because, although it does not happen often, occasional animals react to chemicals, minerals, or nonpathogenic microorganisms in their regular drinking water. Therefore, the regular water supply is discontinued during the food trial period, and only bottled spring or distilled water is used.

All medications are stopped, except those necessary to maintain good health, such as insulin and anticonvulsant drugs. After the 3-day fast, the patient is started on some food that is never, or rarely, eaten, plus peanut, corn or safflower oil, and the owner is instructed to report 3 to 5 days later. To avoid confusion, one should prepare a standard set of instructions, such as in Figure 13–6.

Toys are removed because some toys, especially rubber and soft plastic, may contain chemicals and curing agents that may produce allergic or pseudoallergic reactions. Stuffed toys often contain kapok or other allergenic stuffings, which may produce clinical signs.

Deciding which medications to stop requires good judgment. Obviously, if the patient is subject to epileptiform seizures or requires cardiac drugs or other medication to maintain a reasonable quality of life, these would be continued. If they contain additives, such as preservatives, artificial colors, or flavors to make them palatable, an additive-free dosage form should be sought. On the other hand, palatable vitamins and, in most instances, heartworm medication, can be stopped temporarily without jeopardizing the patient.

The condition does not always improve immediately, even when food allergy is confirmed. Because it can take some time for food residues to be eliminated, a food-trial regimen is followed for at least 3 weeks before one looks for other causes. Even if the patient worsens initially, it does not rule out food allergy. In a condition described in man, "food withdrawal," clinical signs actually become more acute, much like the reaction following narcotic withdrawal, soon after the elimination of an allergenic food. This concept has been the subject of much controversy in human medicine, although similar patterns have been seen in dogs, followed by

INSTRUCTIONS FOR ELIMINATION DIET

1. Administer _____ (tsp.) (tbsp.) of milk of magnesia on the first day of the fast only.
2. Give no food for 3 days. This includes all snacks, tidbits, cookies, and crackers.
3. Give bottled spring water only.
4. Take away all toys.
5. Stop all medications unless instructed otherwise.
6. Observe whether skin condition improves, worsens, or stays the same.
7. If there are other animals in the house, make sure that they also receive the spring water and be sure to feed only when the other dog or cat is out of the house.
8. Be sure that all toilet bowls are covered so the pet does not drink from the toilet, in case he does not like the bottled water.
9. Do not allow the pet out of the house alone, so you can be sure that he does not find and eat something that you do not know about.
10. After 3 days, begin feeding only _____

   plus _____ (tsp.) (tbsp.) salad oil for the next 5 days.
11. Observe whether the skin condition improves, worsens, or remains the same.
12. Call to report on _____
13. If improvement occurs before the end of the 3-day fast, call sooner.

Fig. 13–6.   Instructions for an elimination diet.

gradual improvement as the trial program continues.

If, on the other hand, improvement occurs quickly, before the end of the fast period, no reason exists to continue the fast, and the trial diet can be started sooner.

The principal disadvantages of the 3-day fast and food trial procedure are resistance by the client and improper compliance with the program.

When the client hears that the dog or cat is to be fasted for 3 days, he first blanches and then becomes speechless. One must disarm the client before he has a chance to resist. Before announcing the fast, I always find it useful to tell the client that the procedure is one he will not like, but it will not bother the patient at all. Then, when he blanches, I remind him that I knew he would not like it, but I hasten to reassure him that the pet will be fine and that it is important to determine not only whether food is involved, but to what extent.

If the client does not follow all the instructions for both fasting and food restrictions, it will be difficult to obtain a true evaluation of the extent to which food is involved. It is easy to miss the diagnosis entirely if the client decides that a little of this or that cannot really hurt. Clients should be given written instructions, and they should be admonished to follow them exactly.

A final warning: To avoid facing the issue, clients sometimes ask that the procedure be carried out in the hospital. **This is unequivocally contraindicated.** When diagnostically screening for any allergy problem, it is important that only one change be made at a time. If improvement followed after placing the patient in the hospital, it would be impossible to determine whether the improvement was due to the dietary manipulation or to the change in environment.

The ultimate goal of food trials is to develop a diet that is palatable, nutritious, and nonallergenic. Artificial colors, flavors, and preservatives must be avoided. Therefore, **both the veterinarian and the client must think only in terms of additive-free foods.**

The trial diet should start out with foods that the patient rarely, if ever, eats. Because most pets are fed various forms of canned or packaged pet foods, it is unusual for them to have had fresh cottage cheese, even when fed occasional table scraps. Cottage cheese seems to be well tolerated even in the presence of whole-milk sensitivity or intolerance, and because it is rich in high-quality protein, is easily assimilated, nutritionally sound, and almost completely absorbed, it makes an excellent first food in a trial diet. To supply the unsaturated fats essential to a healthy skin and hair coat, peanut, corn, or safflower oil is added to the cheese. More expensive fatty-acid supplements do little more for the patient than fresh salad oil.

Every 5 days, individual new foods or compatible groups are **added** to the trial diet. One must stress to the client that each new food or group is added to, not substituted in, the diet, to formulate a balanced ration. A first addition to the cottage cheese may be a combination of string beans, peas, and lima beans, for their high protein content and complex carbohydrates. This can be followed by 5 days of chicken and rice. The progression of foods is up to the supervising veterinarian, as long as these foods are additive free and rapidly lead to a balanced diet. A suggested food trial progression follows:

Cottage cheese
String beans, peas, and lima beans
Chicken and rice
Cooked eggs
Potatoes, carrots, and sweet potato or other tuber
Tofu
Banana
Cooked or dry cereals (additive free; read labels)
A vitamin/mineral preparation
Lamb
Fresh fish
Beef or veal
Any other foods, including fruits
During trial diet, cook with bottled spring water and feed the cooking water with its nutritive extracts to the dog or cat

If at any point during the trial diet, one sees an increase or return of clinical signs, that food should be eliminated, and nothing should be fed except foods known to be well tolerated until improvement occurs. On occasion, it may even be necessary to fast the patient again for 1 to 3 days. As soon as improvement occurs, the trial diet continues. If the patient has a reaction to a combined group of foods, then each food must be given separately, to determine which is responsible.

The suspect food is set aside, and after a reasonable period, the patient is again challenged with the food. If the patient has no reaction, the food should now be considered safe and incorporated into the diet. Otherwise, the food is again withheld and fed again at a later time. If a reaction is provoked each of three times, that food should be eliminated completely from the diet.

Regression

Cats show a clinical picture different from dogs, not only in the severity of clinical signs, but in their response to trial diet. In the dog, regression due to exposure to an allergenic food is slowly progressive. The onset of pruritus may be sudden, but it is usually not intense, and the lesions are usually not severe. In the cat, on the other hand, regression is often sudden and explosive, with severe ulcerative lesions recurring almost within hours. One often sees a cat whose lesions have virtually healed regress overnight to its worst state, when it is fed a food to which it is sensitive. Therefore, the clinical course can be much more volatile in the cat than in the dog during the trial-diet period.

The client should keep a diet diary during the trial-diet period (Figure 13–7). The diary can consist of nothing more than a spiral notebook with columns containing the date, foods fed that day, amount and severity of pruritus, if any, presence of gastrointestinal signs, the time of day that reactions occur, and weather conditions. Therefore, if pruritus is variable, one may be able to begin matching good and bad periods with the diet, weather conditions, and other environmental influences. For example, if pruritus is worse or occurs only at certain times of the day, it may be related either to the time of feeding or to a concurrent inhalant allergy, such as molds at night or pollen in the morning and early afternoon. If pruritus is only severe during the day, and especially during good weather, pollens will become a prime suspect. In damp, humid weather, one should suspect molds as contributing factors. None of these suggestions are absolutes, of course, but all help to round out the clinical picture and may help to explain problems that arise during the trial diet.

TREATMENT

The only truly effective treatment is avoidance. Once an allergenic food has been identified, it should be permanently removed from the patient's diet. In man, and occasionally in animals, a tolerance may develop to a formerly allergenic food. Moreover, foods that may cause reactions in large, or frequent, quantities, may be tolerated well in

DIET DIARY

Date	Foods Fed	Amount of Itchiness	Intestinal Problems	Feeding Time	Reaction Time	Weather

Fig. 13–7. Diet diary.

occasional, small doses; however, known allergens should be avoided.

Sensitivities occasionally develop to new foods. Although this does not happen often, it should always be suspected in any animal whose allergy has been under control but suddenly regresses.

Corticosteroids are of limited use in food allergy. In fact, because food allergy is not very responsive to corticosteroids, if the patient has little or no relief following steroid therapy, suspect an underlying food problem. Inhalant allergies, on the other hand, are usually responsive to steroids in the early stages, even though the response often diminishes with time.

Antihistamines give a variable response. In general, they too are of little value in food allergy, although occasional patients respond well.

Immunotherapy also seems to be of little value, for the same reasons discussed under diagnosis.

Urticaria and angioedema require more heroic measures and are treated similarly to anaphylaxis. The preferred procedure is to administer epinephrine and diphenhydramine, as described in Chapter 11. Corticosteroids may be used to control relapses.

Studies on oral cromolyn sodium show this agent to be effective in the prevention of food allergy when the drug is administered regularly before each feeding. Oral cromolyn is not yet readily available in this country, but it would certainly be worth trying in stubborn or resistant cases, when it does become available.

OTHER CONSIDERATIONS IN FOOD ALLERGY

In addition to the role of foods as allergens and their attendant clinical signs, one must also consider their role in the nutrition of the body as a whole, and the skin and hair in particular. Sometimes we forget that skin and hair are composed essentially of protein and, as such, require a good source of high-quality protein if a healthy skin and good coat are to be maintained.

Coupled with this need is the necessity for an adequate supply (up to 18%) of fats in the diet, particularly lineoleic and linolenic acids. Animals deprived of a proper amount of fatty acids develop clinical signs that can easily be confused with allergy, including a dry, itchy skin, erythema, seborrhea, a dry brittle coat, otitis externa, and secondary infections. Therefore, one must thoroughly investigate the patient's diet when evaluating any dermatitis.

Drugs and toxins can cause skin or intestinal changes that may also be confused with allergy. Iodides, for example, can produce a papular eruption over the body. In the days when thallium was a common ingredient in ant traps, occasional animals were poisoned after accidentally eating traps and developed a toxic dermatitis characterized by erythema, epidermal sloughing, and hair loss. I have also seen a case of alopecia and loss of the stratum corneum in a cat, apparently caused by prolonged contact with machine cutting oils.

In addition, malabsorption syndrome (sprue) and Addison's disease, among others, can cause vomiting and diarrhea that may be confused with allergy, if a thorough examination is not made.

Essentially, then, one must not rush into a diagnosis of allergy until a thorough history and physical examination have been completed.

Masking/Unmasking

The concepts of masking/unmasking and latency tolerance that follow are introduced so that the veterinarian reading the human literature will be familiar with them. The processes of masking and unmasking are difficult to understand, but they do have a certain vogue in human medicine and may even have some applicability in veterinary medicine. In "masking," the theory is that subtle food allergy may cause a decrease or abolition of clinical signs following daily ingestion of small amounts of the food to which the patient is allergic. The theory presented to explain the phenomenon suggests that it may be due to a persistent level of protective or blocking antibodies that prevents its identification as an allergen. If the food is not eaten for several days, the allergen is then "unmasked," and clinical signs are seen when the food is next fed.

Latency Tolerance

The concept of "latency tolerance" suggests that a period of time may develop following prolonged avoidance of allergenic foods during which clinical signs will not occur immediately after reintroduction of the food, but such signs will recur after continuous exposure. Therefore, allergy-producing foods may be safely fed, on occasion, following a prolonged period of withdrawal.

Latency tolerance has probably occurred more frequently in dogs and cats than has been recognized. Periodically, a client whose pet's allergy has been under control becomes careless after a period of time and begins feeding allergenic foods. That the patient continues to do well for a while reinforces the client's feeling that the food is no longer a problem. Ultimately, however, unless the dog or cat has actually lost its sensitivity, clinical signs will recur and will continue until the offending food is eliminated.

In summary, we have come a long way in our understanding of food allergy in animals. Much is still unknown, and much of what we do know has been extrapolated from work in man. As increasing numbers of veterinarians become interested in the problem and begin looking for it, however, no doubt our diagnostic and management skills will improve, to the benefit of both the profession and the animals we treat.

REFERENCES

1. Walton, G.S.: Skin responses in the dog and cat to ingested allergens: observations on 100 confirmed cases. Vet. Rec., *81*:709, 1967.
2. Walton, G.S., and Parish, W.E.: Spontaneous allergic dermatitis and enteritis in a cat. Vet. Rec., *83*:35, 1968.
3. Walton, G.S.: Skin manifestation of allergic response in domestic animals. Paper presented at the 85th Annual Congress of the British Veterinary Association, Southport, England, September, 1967.
4. Burns, P.W.: Allergic reactions in dogs. J. Am. Vet. Med. Assoc., *83*:627, 1933.
5. Pomeroy, B.S.: Allergy and allergic skin reactions in the dog. Cornell Vet., *24*:335, 1934.
6. Povar, R.: Food allergy in dogs. J. Am. Vet. Med. Assoc., *110*:61, 1947.
7. Lietze, A.: Laboratory research in food allergy. I. Food allergens. J. Asthma Res., *7*:25, 1969.
8. Wittig, H.J.: Food allergy in children. *In* Current Therapy. Edited by H.F. Conn. Philadelphia, W.B. Saunders, 1973.
9. Thorsen, T.: Relationship of food allergy to feline cystitis. Paper presented at the 29th Annual Meeting of the Academy of Veterinary Allergy, St. Louis, MO, April 10, 1989.
10. Collins, J.: Neurologic manifestations associated with food. Paper presented at the 117th Annual Meeting of the American Veterinary Medicine Association, Washington, D.C., July, 1980.
11. Gelant, S.P., Bullock, J., and Frick, O.L.: An immunological approach to the diagnosis of food sensitivity. Clin. Allergy, *3*:363, 1973.
12. Baker, E.: Food allergy. Vet. Clin. North Am. (Allergy), *4*:79, 1974.

Contact Allergy

Contact allergic dermatitis (CAD) is generally not considered a significant problem in dogs and probably is uncommon in cats, as well. The best-known example in both species is flea-collar dermatitis, especially in the first few years after the introduction of such collars. Considering that CAD does occur, and to a wide range of agents, however, perhaps the problem is more important than was previously thought, or perhaps the wrong diagnostic criteria are applied. Although it is extremely difficult to induce contact allergy artificially wih the classic sensitizers, such as rhus oleoresin, dinitrochlorobenzene (DNCB), or paraphenylenediamine, this difficulty may represent a species-specific variability because neomycin, plastic, and flea-collar sensitivities occur often enough to be a recognizable problem.

The first published case of CAD in domestic animals appeared in 1946 and was of a horse that had been suffering with an unknown dermatitis for 3 years.[1] Lesions were seen over the neck, shoulders, and costal area, locations typically in contact with the leather saddlery. Suspecting a sensitivity to an agent used to treat the leather, the veterinarian conducted patch tests both against the saddle soap and its individual ingredients and against neat's-foot oil, both of which were used on the leather.

Reactions to the saddle soap and neat's-foot oil alone were negative, but when these substances were combined and tested, a 3+ reaction was obtained. When wool yellow dye—used to color the soap—and oil were combined, a 4+ reaction developed. Because the yellow dye alone did not elicit a reaction, the authors concluded that either a chemical reaction occurred between the dye and an impurity in the oil or the oil acted as a vehicle to carry the dye into the dermis.

PATHOPHYSIOLOGY

CAD is a Type IV (cell-mediated, delayed-type) hypersensitivity reaction usually due to simple chemical compounds (haptens) that become allergenic after combining with a protein carrier. When haptens come into intimate contact with the skin, they bind with the dendritic, macrophage-like, immunocompetent Langerhans cells in the skin, cells that "process" the chemicals and "present" them to specific T lymphocytes with receptor sites capable of reacting with the antigen. The T lymphocytes then migrate to the regional lymph nodes, where they undergo further processing and produce large numbers of antigen-specific T-effector cells and memory cells, which then enter the circulation and go on "immune surveillance patrol." Future contact with the antigen creates an antigenic focus that the specifically sensitized lymphocytes attempt to destroy. It is this reaction that results in CAD.

Histologically, one may see vasodilation and perivascular round-cell infiltration, as well as infiltration with polymorphonuclear cells, monocytes, and eosinophils.

Experimentally, contact sensitivity is extremely difficult to induce. In one report, dogs sensitized to DNCB, a potent sensitizer, developed reactions that were much milder than those seen in either guinea pigs or man.[2] In experiments using up to 5% poison ivy extract, the results were much more variable and inconclusive.

CAD can be experimentally induced in the cat, on the other hand, as demonstrated by Schultz and Maguire, using DNCB.[3] Sensitization was induced in the animals' interscapular skin, and the ear was used for challenge. Sensitized cats showed a significant difference in pinnal thickness, as compared to nonsensitized or vehicle-challenged cats, and the histopathologic features were consistent with CAD.

Hair is a good natural barrier to contact allergens, so naturally occurring reactions are seen mostly on hairless or thin-haired areas of the skin or between the foot pads. Haired areas of the skin can become involved, as in flea-collar dermatitis, if the contactant is either in solution, or a vapor, ensuring adequate, continuous skin exposure. When the resins in pollen grains or in cut vegetation, such as mowed grass, are in intimate contact with the interdigital spaces of the foot pads, these substances can cause contact sensitivity of the feet.

ETIOLOGIC AGENTS

The problem with listing etiologic agents is that, in spite of the difficulty with which CAD can be induced experimentally in the dog, presumptive, spontaneous cases resulting from exposure to poison ivy, poison oak, jasmine, and other plant material have been reported.[4,5] Most reported patients were not challenged by patch testing, although clinically, the lesions flared with exposure to, and cleared on withdrawal of, the suspect allergen.

Drugs and chemicals have also been reported to be contact allergens. These substances include such commonly used agents as penicillin, neomycin, tetracaine and related compounds, insecticides, particularly flea collars and medallions, coal-tar products, and perfumes. Formaldehyde, an important contact sensitizer for man, is used in the manufacture or surface treatment of many household products and plastics. One of the most common household sources of formaldehyde, and one that causes problems in man, are facial tissues treated with the chemical to give them body. Formaldehyde has not yet been reported as a problem in dogs and cats, but it and all sensitizing chemical compounds should be considered potential problems for pets.

Certain heavy metals have caused a reaction in animals, especially on the thin-coated portion of the ventral neck. Nickel or chrome steel license or other identification tags are the most serious offenders in this regard because they are in constant contact with a limited portion of the body.

Synthetic fibers, such as nylon and Dacron, are not generally considered allergenic, but the dyes and dyeing process can cause CAD. This problem largely depends on whether the dye is incorporated into the synthetic fiber, in which case it is generally inert, or applied to the surface of the fiber, such as in the pattern dyeing of rugs. Surface dyes allow direct contact of the dye with the skin and increase the potential for an allergic response.

Soft plastic or rubber has also been incriminated in contact allergy; the best-known example is the dermatitis occasionally seen around the face or muzzle of some dogs eating from soft rubber or soft plastic bowls. Lesions can become extremely inflamed and ulcerative and must be differentiated from immune-mediated disease or even cancer.

ALLERGY VERSUS IRRITATION

CAD must be differentiated from contact irritation, which can be caused by caustic irritants, abrasive compounds, soaps, disinfectants, cleaning agents, petroleum compounds, organic solvents, and any other potentially irritative material or chemical compound. The reaction is due specifically to the irritating effects of the contactant and has no immune basis. Because some compounds can act as both irritants and sensitizers, and because clinical signs are often similar, distinguishing between the two by examination alone is not always easy. In some instances, the patient's history helps to make the diagnosis, whereas in others, biopsies may be required.

Overbathing is an occasional cause of contact irritation resulting in a dry, scaling skin. Some dogs also have a severe, acute dermatitis as a result of their owners applying household cleaning agents to the animals' skin. I vividly remember a hound presented for examination with an acutely inflamed skin, patchy hair loss, and exfoliative dermatitis. The owner had decided that because pine-tar disinfectant solution was doing such a good job in his home, it ought to be great on his dog. Fortunately, the dog recovered quickly following warm water soaks and corticosteroids.

Even bland soaps can cause contact irritation of the skin, and particularly the scrotum, if they are not thoroughly rinsed from the coat.

CLINICAL SIGNS

Because of the protective barrier provided by the coat, lesions are usually limited to the thin-haired or hairless regions of the body, such as the lower abdomen and ventral surface, muzzle, lips, volar webbing of the feet, medial pinnae, and ear canals. Lesions are not characteristic and can vary from mild to severe, depending on the length of contact and the potency of the sensitizer.

Even though both CAD and other forms of allergic dermatitis may exhibit a papular eruption, scales, crusts, seborrhea, and erosions, fine vesiculation is more likely to develop with CAD than with food or allergic inhalant dermatitis. One difference frequently seen with CAD is slow resolution of the dermal lesions when compared to the other types of allergic dermatitis.

With other forms of allergic skin disease, the skin begins to clear within hours of removing the offending food or inhalant. In fact, I frequently examine patients with minimal lesions, only to have clients tell me that, just hours before, the skin had been "a bloody mess." In CAD, on the other hand, lesions may heal slowly, sometimes taking weeks to clear. Severely erosive lesions of flea-collar dermatitis, for example, have persisted for 4 weeks or longer after removal of the collar before they finally disappear.

Lesions also vary based on location and etiologic agent. For example, the basic location of flea-collar dermatitis is the neck, with satellite lesions extending in either direction toward the head or shoulders. Initially, the lesions consist of an erythematous ring around the neck that is more severe on the dorsal aspect where the collar lies in more intimate contact with the neck. If the collar is not removed, the condition may progress to scaling, crusts, and eventual ulcerations, until an erosive ring develops around the neck. These lesions may take weeks to heal, possibly because of antigen bound to skin protein and released slowly.

Plastic/rubber food-bowl dermatitis classically affects the lips, nose, and muzzle (Fig. 14–1), but it may also affect the paws if the feet are in contact with the bowl while the animal eats. Characteristically, the lesions on

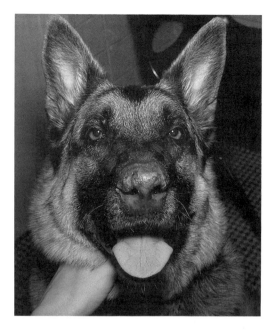

Fig. 14–1. Plastic/rubber food-bowl dermatitis in a German shepherd.

the face are limited to the area in contact with the bowl and may even be sharply demarcated to conform to the rim. Lesions can become severe, but once the bowl is removed, they begin to clear and usually disappear within a few weeks.

Metal CAD often goes unrecognized or is ascribed to other causes. Identification tags are the most common metallic allergen. The key here is that the lesions are concentrated in the area where the metal tags hang on the ventral neck, usually between the larynx and the thoracic inlet (Fig. 14–2). Lesions are characterized by loss of hair, lichenification, thickening of the skin, and pigmentation, usually without much of an acute inflammatory reaction. Here, too, resolution of the lesions can be slow following removal of the tags.

Certain medications have also been incriminated in the induction of contact allergy when they are applied topically for prolonged periods of time. The principal agents of interest in veterinary medicine are neomycin, a popular antibiotic found in several topical preparations, and tetracaine and other related topical local anesthetics. Although any area of the body treated with sensitizing compounds can develop lesions, the

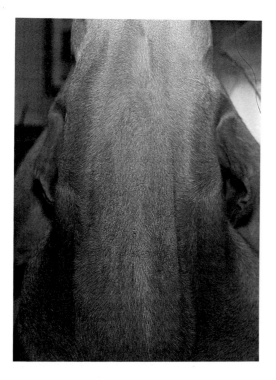

Fig. 14–2. Metal-contact allergic dermatitis.

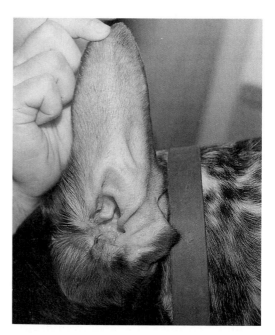

Fig. 14–3. Medication-associated contact allergic dermatitis of the ear in a German short-haired pointer.

ear canal and pinna seem to be the most common sites for medication-associated CAD (Fig. 14–3). Whether this predisposition represents a specific increased sensitivity of otic tissues or increased exposure because of the frequency of recurrent otitis and the number of topical ear preparations containing antibiotics and topical anesthetics is uncertain. Affected tissues become inflamed and edematous and may become ulcerated.

Typically, patients with otitis that are treated with sensitizing compounds seem to improve initially, only to regress as treatment continues. Because of the initial improvement, the clinician often thinks that additional medication is needed, and treatment is continued, initiating an ever-worsening condition. In another situation, patients are treated for otitis, the condition clears, and otitis recurs later. Because the tissue has become sensitized by the earlier treatment, reinstitution of the medication often results in CAD and a rapidly worsening clinical response. Fortunately, discontinuing medication is curative, and unlike in some other contact sensitivities, response is usually rapid and complete. A good rule of thumb is

to suspect CAD in any skin condition that regresses after initial improvement while the patient is receiving topical therapy, especially if either the vehicle or the active ingredient is a known contact sensitizer.

Dyes, particularly those used on carpets, generally affect the ventral surface and interdigital webbing of the volar surfaces of patients' feet. Little can be done except to remove the carpet from the dog or the dog from the carpet.

Often overlooked causes of CAD are carpet fresheners and deodorizers. These substances can cause intense pruritus. Although lesions such as erythema, papules, pustules, and crusts are usually found (Fig. 14–4), the only clinical sign may be pruritus. A recent case report describing lesions associated with a carpet freshener demonstrated that patch testing can be of value in making a positive diagnosis.[6]

DIAGNOSIS

Because lesions are not specifically characteristic, CAD can easily be confused with food and inhalant allergy, contact irritation, and other skin problems. The distribution of lesions can be helpful in making a diagnosis

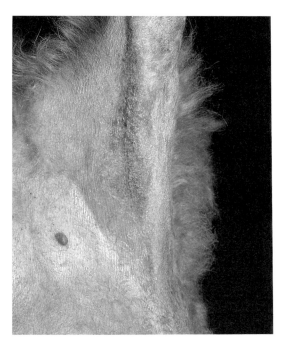

Fig. 14–4. Contact allergic dermatitis caused by a carpet freshener in a poodle.

because contact sensitivity usually occurs on the thin-haired areas of the body, such as the volar surfaces of the feet, the axillae, the muzzle, and the lower abdomen. In fact, lesions may be pronounced on a bare, exposed area of the skin, only to stop abruptly at the hair line. Do not assume, however, that lesions are not present on the haired skin just because they are not obvious. A wide patch of hair surrounding the lesion should always be removed, and the exposed skin should be examined to be sure that lesions are not there. The patient's history also plays an important role in diagnosis, especially as it relates to the pet's environment, contactants, and habits.

Biopsy is of little diagnostic help, except possibly to rule out other conditions.

If one suspects that a contact sensitivity has developed to a sensitizer indigenous to the pet's household, such as a carpet freshener or dye, a presumptive diagnosis often can be made based on the distribution of lesions and an environmental history. In such cases, the pet is removed from its normal environment by being placed in a boarding kennel, hospital, or another home. If the lesions improve or clear after a reasonable period of time, the patient is returned to its normal environment and is observed for recurrence of clinical signs. This diagnostic procedure is not nearly as effective for the identification of CAD as it is in the diagnosis of environmental inhalant allergies, but it can be used where patch testing is not practical or feasible. The principal criteria for differentiating between CAD and AID is that AID patients recover rapidly following removal from the offending allergen, whereas patients with CAD take much longer to respond.

The only diagnostic test of value is the patch test, which, as can be imagined, is not easy to perform in the dog and cat. When specific chemicals or other agents are suspected allergens, one should affix cotton or other suitable pads impregnated with the test materials to the patient's shaved skin for up to 72 hours. The test sites are read every 24 hours, and if erythema, vesicles, papules, or other eruptions are seen, the test is considered positive and is discontinued. If the test site remains negative after 72 hours, the result is considered negative.

The major problem in patch testing is applying the patches so they are comfortable, are not removed by the patient, and do not shift or slip. Unless the patch remains in constant contact with the test site, it is unreliable. The best way to proceed is to shave a patch of skin along the dorsolateral aspect of the patient's trunk or thorax, bind it to the skin with stretch bandage, and tape the whole area with elastic tape. This procedure is obviously not easy, especially if the site is to be examined daily.

TREATMENT

The treatment of choice, as with all allergy, is avoidance. In the acute stages, however, it is often beneficial to administer intralesional or sublesional injections of a short- or intermediate-acting corticosteroid. Topical steroids also offer some relief. Because the reaction is cell mediated, little, if any, benefit can be expected from either antihistamines or immunotherapy. Response to treatment can be slow, and treatments should be repeated as needed.

Finally, a diagnosis of contact allergy does not preclude the presence of other concurrent problems, such as dermatophytosis, atopic dermatitis, and pyoderma. Therefore, one should keep an open mind in evaluating unresponsive patients or those responding slowly to treatment. Both the patient and the diagnosis should be re-evaluated, and either a more accurate diagnosis should be made or other possible concurrent problems should be considered.

REFERENCES

1. Reddin, L., and Stever, D.W.: Allergic contact dermatitis in the horse. North Am. Vet., *27*:561, 1946.
2. Schultz, K.T., and Maguire, H.C.: Chemically induced delayed hypersensitivity in the dog. Vet. Immunol. Immunopathol., *3*:585, 1982.
3. Gaafar, S.M., and Krawiec, D.R.: Chemical sensitizers and contact dermatitis. Am. Anim. Hosp. Assoc., *10*:133, 1974.
4. Ripps, J.H.: Allergic dermatitis in a dog. J. Am. Vet. Med. Assoc., *133*:479, 1958.
5. Muller, B.H.: Contact dermatitis in animals. Arch. Dermatol., *96*:423, 1967.
6. Comer, K.M.: Carpet deodorizer as a contact allergen in a dog. J. Am. Vet. Med. Assoc., *193*:1553, 1988.

COLOR PLATES

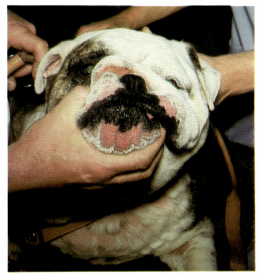

Fig. 5–1. Allergic erythema around the muzzle of an English bulldog.

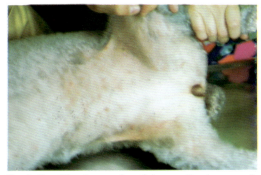

Fig. 5–2. Allergic papulonodular eruption in a poodle.

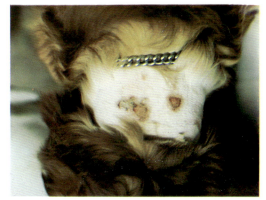

Fig. 5–4. Allergic exudative dermatitis in a golden retriever.

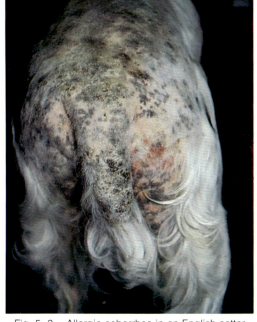

Fig. 5–3. Allergic seborrhea in an English setter.

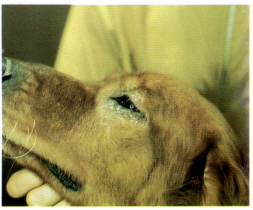

Fig. 5–5. Allergic periorbital alopecia in a golden retriever.

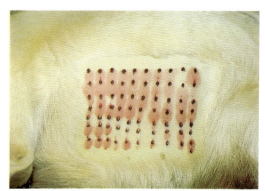

Fig. 10–8. Positive skin-test reaction in the dog. (Courtesy of Dr. John M. MacDonald, Auburn University School of Veterinary Medicine, Auburn, Alabama.)

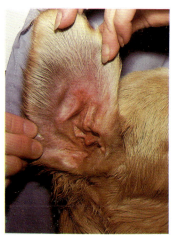

Fig. 5–6. Allergic otitis in a golden retriever.

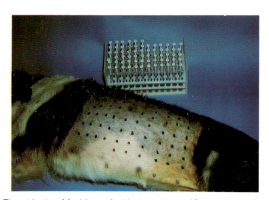

Fig. 10–1. Marking of skin-test sites. (Courtesy of Dr. John M. MacDonald, Auburn University School of Veterinary Medicine, Auburn, Alabama.)

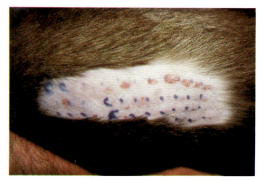

Fig. 10–6. Positive skin-test reaction in the dog.

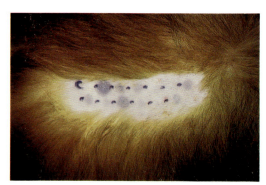

Fig. 10–9. Positive skin-test reaction in the dog as evidenced by blue dye.

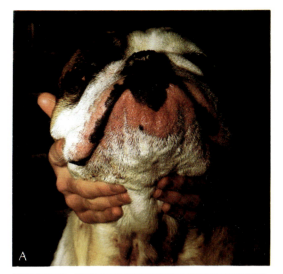

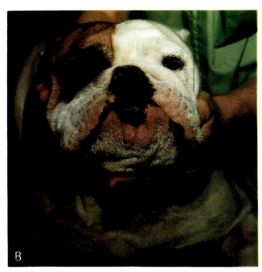

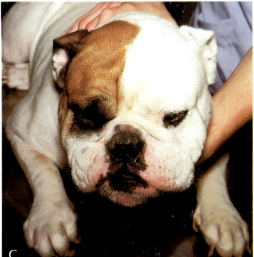

Fig. 11–1.   Seasonal allergic dermatitis in an English bull-dog during a course of immunotherapy. *A,* Condition before therapy. *B* and *C,* Visible improvements 1 and 2 months, respectively, after beginning therapy.

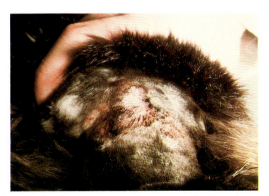

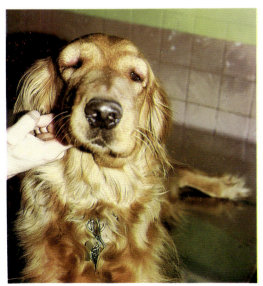

Fig. 13–1.   Severe allergic dermatitis with alopecia and ulceration.

Fig. 13–2.   Allergic urticaria and angioedema in a golden retriever.

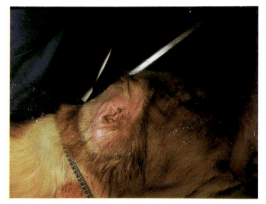

Fig. 13–3. Allergic otitis with pinnal erythema and edema in a golden retriever.

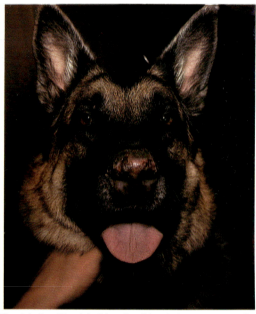

Fig. 14–1. Plastic/rubber food-bowl dermatitis in a German shepherd.

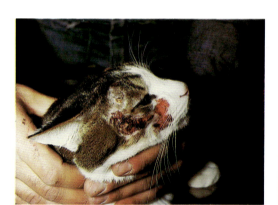

Fig. 13–4. Ulcerative allergic dermatitis in a cat.

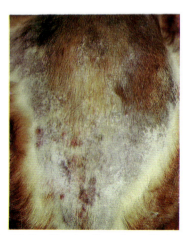

Fig. 13–5. Allergic miliary dermatitis in a cat.

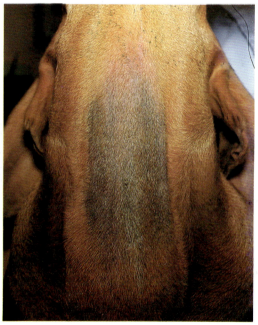

Fig. 14–2. Metal-contact allergic dermatitis.

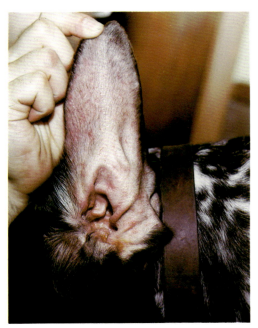

Fig. 14–3. Medication-associated contact allergic dermatitis of the ear in a German short-haired pointer.

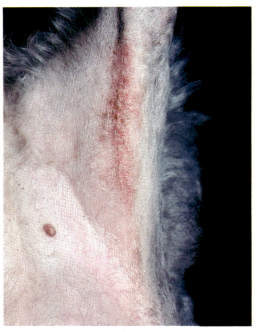

Fig. 14–4. Contact allergic dermatitis caused by a carpet freshener in a poodle.

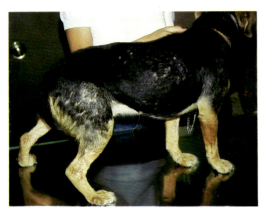

Fig. 16–1. Bacterial dermatitis.

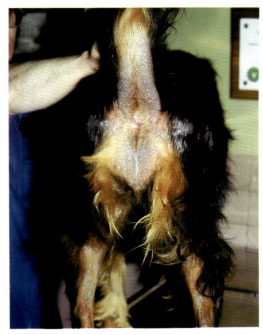

Fig. 16–2. Dermatitis in a dog with anal sac infection.

15 || *Insect Hypersensitivity*

Insects exist in both free-living and parasitic forms, each of which is capable of eliciting hypersensitivity responses. With most parasitic forms, the reaction develops in response to salivary allergens injected while the insect is taking a blood meal. A much smaller number, however, live within body tissues, in which case the host becomes sensitized to the parasite's excrement or other metabolites. Even though the free-living forms do not depend on a living host for their existence, severe, even life-threatening, reactions have been caused by venoms injected during attacks by stinging insects. Other nonvenomous, free-living insects such as sand flies, mayflies, and cockroaches have been responsible for allergic reactions, including asthma, in man. Such reactions can be caused by fine, hair-like filaments, body fragments, and excrement.

Even though accurate incidence figures are not available, the flea alone could easily be counted as the major potential insect sensitizer in both dogs and cats. To this can be added such common parasites as demodex and sarcoptes, less allergenic parasites such as ticks, lice, and chiggers, and the free-living insects, including the ubiquitous house dust mite (considered by many to be the most significant component of house dust), the stinging insects of the Hymenoptera order (bees, yellow jackets, wasps, and hornets), mosquitoes, fire ants, and stable flies.

The common bond among stinging, biting, sucking, or burrowing insects is their ability to stimulate an immune response. Although both Type I and Type IV reactions can be induced, especially to fleas, the immunoglobulin E (IgE)-mediated immediate reactions are by far the more significant and destructive. Type I reactions are typically pruritic and can be intense, resulting in scratching, biting, chewing, and self-mutilation. This dual immune response may represent the ontogenic progression of immunity in that, in some instances, such as flea-bite-induced sensitivity,[1] the cell-mediated response is seen first, and the immediate type follows several weeks later. A similar response also often occurs in bacterial sensitivity, particularly following staphylococcal infection.[2] The basic immune response to nonbiting insects, such as house dust mite and cockroach, on the other hand, in which sensitivity is caused by inhaled body fragments, is a Type I, immediate reaction.

FLEAS

The pathogenesis of flea-bite allergy is still obscure and confusing, even though it has been extensively investigated over the years. Until recently, it was thought that fleas, in sufficient concentration, would cause either an allergic reaction or an irritation. As a corollary, it was further reasoned that the larger the number of fleas, and the longer the contact with the patient, the more likely the development of either irritation or allergy, and the worse it would become. These theories are now seriously questioned. Because some dogs and many cats can harbor fleas, and sometimes in large numbers, without obvious skin lesions, it is becoming increasingly apparent that flea-infested patients either develop a flea-bite allergy or remain asymptomatic. Further, studies over the past few years have suggested that flea-allergic dogs, when left untreated to cope with their fleas, gradually lose their sensitivity.

Apparently, flea-bite allergy occurs in two stages, and this process is also difficult to explain. Because salivary antigens, like other insect venoms and salivary antigens, are incomplete, thereby acting as haptens, the initial response to fleas is a Type IV, cell-mediated reaction. In spite of the haptenic saliva, an immediate, Type I reaction develops within weeks, contrary to what one would ordinarily expect. In addition to the immediate and delayed hypersensitivities, evidence also suggests that cutaneous basophil hypersensitivity plays a role in the development of flea-bite allergy.[3] To complicate matters further, studies at the University of Florida suggest that if the dog is left untreated, and if fleas are allowed to accumulate on the dog, the sensitivity will gradually disappear; this finding suggests that a state of tolerance may develop. This would certainly make sense in nature because one doubts whether the species could survive for long in the wild, if all its time and energy were spent scratching at fleas. From a human point of view, we could not accept coexistence with fleas; not only are they an irritative nuisance, but also they are serious disease carriers. From the dog's point of view, however, we may be changing their resistance to render them increasingly intolerant of a flea infestation.

Some dogs, and probably some cats, seem to have an innate resistance, or biochemical difference, making them unattractive to fleas. In one dog colony used for studying flea infestations, in which the dogs were allowed to mingle freely, some dogs consistently had high numbers of fleas ranging from hundreds to a thousand or more, whereas others rarely had as many as fifty. This situation is probably like that in man, where of a group sitting on a warm summer's eve, some are literally eaten alive by mosquitoes, whereas others rarely sustain a bite.

The cat seems to be an excellent example of natural tolerance to fleas. No incidence figures exist for the number of cats actually infested with fleas relative to the number showing signs of allergic flea-bite dermatitis. Yet experience makes one conclude that the number of flea-infested cats that actually show clinical signs must be small.

One of the factors complicating a determination in the dog is that the skin is not usually searched for fleas unless the dog is scratching. The first signs of "flea-bite dermatitis" often coincide with the onset of the principal inhalant allergy season. For many dogs, this season is usually August through October. The client brings in a dog that is scratching and has an inflamed skin, a flea is seen, and obviously, the problem must be due to fleas. Flea treatment is given, and if no improvement occurs, the logical conclusion is that the dog must still have fleas, even if they cannot be found. Therefore, treatment is intensified and continued until the end of the allergy season, when the fleas "miraculously" disappear.

Because these dogs were not examined before their skin problems began, one has no way of knowing how long they had been infested with fleas. Yet if these same dogs were searched earlier in the season, there is no doubt that many would harbor fleas without problems. Such an observation suggests three possibilities: (1) the dog does not have flea-allergy dermatitis, but is really suffering from allergic inhalant dermatitis; (2) the flea bites are acting as "loading factors" because of a low-grade sensitivity, increasing the severity of the inhalant dermatitis; or (3) both flea-allergic and allergic inhalant dermatitis are present.

Diagnosis

Diagnosis is based on finding fleas or "flea dirt" (excrement), eliminating the fleas, and looking for improvement. When only a few fleas are present, they may be difficult to find, in which case a flea comb can be useful. If you see dark particles, but you are not certain whether they are actually flea dirt, place a few specks on a white paper towel or other white surface, put a drop of water on it, and because it contains a high quantity of hemoglobin as a result of the fleas' blood-feeding habits, look for the red pigment to "bleed" out of the "dirt."

Intradermal flea antigen is also a useful diagnostic tool. Properly administered, it can help you to identify those animals actually allergic to fleas, not only to confirm the diagnosis, but also to present visual evidence of flea-bite sensitivity and, one hopes, to encourage the client to be meticulous in maintaining a good flea-control program. **It is important to use only nonglycerinated test extracts because even small amounts of glycerin can cause an irritative, false-positive response.** Remember also that negative reactions do not rule out flea-allergic dermatitis; both false-positive and false-negative reactions can occur. Finally, the best diagnostic proof is to eliminate the fleas and look for improvement.

Management

The most effective treatment for flea-bite dermatitis is the elimination of fleas, both on the patient and in the environment. Unfortunately, this is easier said than done. Eliminating fleas is not as difficult in the northern part of the country, or in desert areas with low humidity, as in the rest of the country. In those vast regions where the winters are mild and the rest of the year is warm and humid, however, fleas can be virtually impossible to control.

Every veterinarian has his favorite parasiticide, and both the patient and premises should be treated regularly. **ALWAYS FOLLOW PACKAGE INSTRUCTIONS.**

Flea collars are an open question. Although newer formulations seem to have reduced the number of flea-collar dermatitides in recent years, these reactions still do occur. Moreover, in spite of data showing efficacy for up to 11 months with some flea collars, most seem to lose effectiveness quickly.

As adjunctive therapy, studies at the University of Florida demonstrated that Avon's Skin-So-Soft was effective in repelling and reducing, but not eliminating, flea populations on dogs,[4] when the lotion is applied as a dip or sponged on at a concentration of 1.5 oz/gal water and used as necessary. The Skin-So-Soft can also be added to flea dipping solutions. As for electronic flea collars, definite recommendations cannot be made at this time. Some evidence suggests that the collars substantially reduce the numbers of fleas on animals, but do not eliminate them. I have clients who think these collars are wonderful, and others who think they are worthless. Others have told me that one brand did not work, but when they switched to another, it seemed to work well. Whether this difference is due to a different electronic frequency, a reduction in overall environmental flea population, or the client's imagination is hard to say.

DEMODEX

For all the vast increase in knowledge of the pathogenesis and immunobiology of demodicosis in recent years, the disease still remains difficult and troubling. That a genetic predisposition exists is without doubt. Certainly, alterations of the immune system also play a role, as evidenced by the increased incidence of demodicosis among animals immunosuppressed by drugs, age, tumors, or liver disease. Immune mechanisms in the pathogenesis of this disease are still not totally clear, but the consensus is that cell-mediated immunity apparently plays an important role in controlling demodex and in preventing infection in normal dogs.

Immune Reactions

Once demodex is established, colonization of the hair follicles leads to disruption and destruction of the follicle with hair loss, folliculitis, furunculosis, and spread of disease. Earlier studies suggested that the principal immune response was a Type IV reaction, which may either represent a contact-type sensitivity due to the presence of somatic particles or of metabolites in contact with the epidermal Langerhans' cells or a foreign-body reaction due to the mass of parasites localized in the follicles, or both. These studies are now questioned, so the significance of the work and of its conclusions is uncertain.

A Type I reaction is considered relatively unimportant in the clinical response, but this assessment is also open to question because histamine has been found in high levels in the skin of dogs with demodicosis. In fact, in my studies, areas of clinically active invasion could be outlined by the blue hue that developed following the intravenous administration of trypan blue or Evans blue dyes, a finding suggesting edema caused by histamine or other inflammatory mediators. In addition, although a cell-mediated immune response may be the cause of both the inflammation and pruritus frequently seen in this disease, the degree of erythema and pruritus in some cases suggests that these reactions are probably Type I, rather than Type IV.

A secondary immune response to severe demodicosis is the development of a serum immunosuppressive factor that suppresses T-cell blastogenesis responses. This factor disappears as dogs respond to therapy. It is tempting to speculate whether serum plasmapheresis would be of value in the therapy of severe, unresponsive disease.

Treatment

Parasiticidal Treatment

Treatment depends not only on the use of parasiticides, such as amitraz, but also on the general health of the patient and the condition of the immune system.

Nonspecific Treatment

Patients should be placed on a nutritious diet with high-quality protein and optimum fatty-acid and vitamin/mineral supplementation. In addition, good grooming on a daily basis is essential for a healthy skin and hair coat.

Vitamin E

A report at the annual meeting of the Academy of Veterinary Dermatology several years ago suggested that an excellent therapeutic response could be expected with the administration of 200 IU of vitamin E five times daily. The results of my clinical trials were equivocal, at best, although some cases did seem to respond more quickly than would have been expected. Fortunately, this vitamin is tolerated well and rarely has side effects, so it is certainly worth trying as part of your treatment regimen. Although the original investigator specified 200 IU five times daily, no rational explanation exists for dividing the dose, so I see no reason that 1000 IU once daily or 500 IU twice daily cannot be given.

Immunostimulants

The only immunostimulant I have found of value in the treatment of demodex is staphylococcus toxoid. I and others have tried levamisole, with poor or no response. Because this drug is potentially toxic, and is of no value for the treatment of demodex, it should not be used. Staphylococcus toxoid, on the other hand, has a nonspecific stimulatory effect on cell-mediated immunity and has helped to shorten treatment time and to relieve the acute stage of the disease in many

Table 15–1. Dosage Schedule for Staphylococcal Toxoid

Dose No.	Amount (ml)	Dose No.	Amount (ml)
1	0.25	5	1.25
2	0.50	6	1.50
3	0.75	7	1.75
4	1.00	8	2.00

cases. For maximum therapeutic effect, it must be used properly. My personal preference is for Staphoid A-B (Coopers-Pitman Moore), administered in an 8-dose series. The first 5 doses are given every day, or as close to daily as possible, and the last 3 doses are given 1 week apart. Starting with 0.25 ml, each dose is increased by 0.25 ml until a total of 2 ml is given at the eighth injection (Table 15–1). Most important is to divide the dose into 3 portions, so 0.1 ml is always given intradermally, and the balance is split, with half given subcutaneously and the balance given intramuscularly.

SARCOPTES AND NOTOEDRES

Reaction in the skin to these and other burrowing parasites, such as creeping eruption of hookworm larvae and pelodera (rhabditic) dermatitis, is twofold: (1) an inflammatory response is caused by the direct mechanical effect of burrowing and tissue destruction; and (2) a foreign-body reaction, with its accompanying cell-mediated immune response, is directed against the parasite, its excrement, and other metabolites and body fragments.

In the early developmental phase, lesions may be minimal, even though pruritus can be intense. At this stage, it is necessary to search carefully to find inflammatory papules, nodules, or crusts. As the condition progresses, erythema becomes pronounced and diffuse, and the pruritus intensifies. In the later stages, one sees severe hair loss, thickening of the skin, scales, crusts, and ulcerations.

Diagnosis is based on finding the parasite, its eggs, or excrement in skin scrapings. They are not always easy to find, especially if corticosteroids have been used to control itching. The most productive place to scrape is the ear margins, although mites are often found in any crusting area of the body. If lesions are minimal, or if they are not pronounced, carefully palpate the patient's ear margins for small scaling patches or crusts, which should then be scraped deeply. Rolling the ear between the fingers generally initiates a scratch reflex, which, although not pathognomonic for mange, should make one suspicious.

Fortunately, once the diagnosis is made, the parasite is usually susceptible to most acaricidal preparations.

BITING INSECTS

Into this category are lumped such diverse insect pests and parasites as biting flies, mosquitoes, ticks, biting and sucking lice, chiggers, cheyletiella, and fleas, although fleas constitute a problem serious enough to be discussed separately. Here, too, the binding thread is the induction of an immune response, with the Type I, immediate reaction the most important clinically. Such reactions occur within minutes and are typified by the inflamed, pruritic, hive-like lesions produced by the bites of these insects.

In addition to the immune response induced by their bite, the saliva of many of these parasites contains vasoactive amines, anticoagulants, and irritants capable of causing a nonspecific inflammatory reaction characterized by a stinging sensation and a zone of inflammation around the bite. The intensity of the reaction usually subsides quickly, although itching may continue for 24 hours or longer.

Fortunately, many animals are apparently resistant, not only to the insects themselves, but also to the effects of their bites. In animals that are not so lucky, however, insect repellents are often effective in driving off flies and mosquitoes. If bites are severe enough, one should shave the lesions and apply a sodium bicarbonate paste, calamine lotion, a 1% topical hydrocortisone preparation, or a topical anesthetic.

Ticks, lice, chiggers, pelodera, and cheyletiella are easily removed from the body by insecticidal dips. Solitary ticks can be removed by first coating them with a drop of oil or an insecticide, then waiting about 5 minutes, and finally grasping the tick's head with tweezers or forceps and gently easing it out of the patient's skin. If the tick's body is grasped and yanked, the head may be left behind in the skin and may then cause a foreign-body reaction that could take a week or longer to resolve. The habit of grasping the tick and crushing it between the fingers should be discouraged because tick-borne diseases, including Lyme disease, can be transmitted in this way.

HYMENOPTERA

Bees, wasps, hornets, and yellow jackets do not represent a major serious threat to dogs, although acute anaphylactic, and even fatal, reactions have been reported. I know of no reports of such reactions in cats. Dense fur is obviously protective; stinging insects have a difficult time penetrating the skin, except in thinly coated areas. In man, the potential for fatal and near-fatal reactions is so serious that sensitive individuals are advised to carry syringes of epinephrine with them for emergencies.

The principal immune response is an immediate, Type I, local or systemic anaphylactic reaction, with clinical signs ranging from localized swelling to collapse.

The first published report of anaphylaxis in a dog of which I am aware was by a physician/allergist who was called to see a neighbor's German shepherd, which was in a state of near collapse. The dog had been stung by a bee and within minutes began showing signs of distress. The closest veterinarian was too far away to render the type of emergency service required because the physician thought it appeared to be life-threatening. The allergist therefore treated it as he would any human patient, with epinephrine and antihistamines. Fortunately, the dog responded quickly, and recovery was uneventful.

The bee's stinger is a modified ovipositor, and only the female stings. Except for the honeybee, all other important members of this group attack their victim, inject their venom, and withdraw the stinger. The honeybee is unique in that it has barbs on the end of its stinger that prevent its withdrawal, thus tearing out the venom sac as the bee flies away to die. Meanwhile, the sac continues to pump venom into the skin for at least several minutes. Therefore, every effort should be made to remove the stinger as quickly as possible, to minimize the amount of venom injected.

Prevention is much better than treatment, and as with other allergens, the best prevention is avoidance. Although wasps, hornets, and bees build aerial nests attached to the eaves of buildings or tree branches, the ill-tempered yellow jackets build their nests underground in tall grass, under rocks, or around building foundations. It is almost impossible to keep dogs from rooting in flower and shrubbery beds or from disturbing the underground yellow jacket nests, but one can avoid the use of doggy "colognes" or other aromatic preparations that attract stinging insects. If the patient is particularly sensitive to Hymenoptera stings, and they occur in spite of preventive measures, treatment with the newer specific venom or mixed Hymenoptera antigens seem to work well in either preventing or minimizing reactions. A number of my canine patients had histories of severe reactions to Hymenoptera stings characterized by swelling, vomiting, and occasional respiratory distress. Following immunotherapy, several owners reported that the dogs had subsequently been stung, but the ensuing reaction was reduced. Because we have neither a specific veterinary product nor a recommended dosage schedule for dogs, we must use human products and follow the schedule recommended for man.

REFERENCES

1. Tizard, I.: Veterinary Immunology: An Introduction, 3rd Ed. Philadelphia, W.B. Saunders, 1987.
2. Rajka, G.: Studies in hypersensitivity to molds and staphylococci in prurigo Besnier (atopic dermatitis). Acta Derm. Venereol. (Stockholm), *43 (Suppl. 54)*:43, 1963.
3. Halliwell, R.E.W., and Schemmer, K.R.: The role of basophils in the immunopathogenesis of hypersensitivities to fleas (Ctenocephalides felis) in dogs. Vet. Immunol. Immunopathol., *15*:203, 1987.
4. Fehrer, S.L., and Halliwell, R.E.: Effectiveness of Avon's Skin-So-Soft as a flea repellent on dogs. J. Am. Anim. Hosp. Assoc., *23*:217, 1987.

Staphylococcal Sensitivity and Anal Sac Disease

STAPHYLOCOCCAL SENSITIVITY

Bacterial sensitivity is probably one of the most controversial subjects in veterinary allergy and dermatology. No uniformity exists for specific diagnostic criteria, and all veterinarians do not necessarily agree on just what constitutes this troublesome syndrome. All the foregoing notwithstanding, there is consensus on at least part of this clinical entity: patients have a history of current or prior bacterial infection, lesions are discrete, although they may coalesce, and pruritus is present. Some general consensus also suggests that most clinical bacterial sensitivity is due to staphylococci, with occasional cases due to streptococci or other bacteria.

Immunology

Bacteria are virtually multiple-antigen production plants, because even simple bacteria produce an assortment of antigens derived from the complex molecules of their cell wall, as well as the exotoxins produced in the wall of gram-negative bacteria. In addition, some bacteria produce endotoxins, necrotoxins, assorted lysins and hemolysins, and a variety of other metabolic products, all of which can be antigenic. Staphylococci, probably the most important group of bacteria in the induction of hypersensitivity, produce a host of antigens, including cell-wall antigens, exotoxins, assorted hemolysins, and lysins.

Although bacteria can elicit Type I, III, and IV immune responses, the Type I and IV reactions are of most interest to the allergist. Just as immunoglobulin M (IgM), the more primitive antibody response, precedes the production of more specific IgG as a response to bacteria, a Type IV, teleologically older, cell-mediated immune reaction often precedes the onset of the immediate (Type I) response. This pattern has been amply demonstrated in an extensive series of experi-

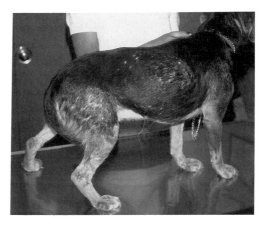

Fig. 16–1. Bacterial dermatitis.

ments with both streptococcus and staphylococcus.

Clinical Signs

Clinically, lesions vary from patient to patient, although I have had a strong impression over the years that shepherd-type dogs have a more specific syndrome. In these dogs, one usually sees erythema, alopecia, crusting, and ulceration, and lesions are localized primarily around the hindquarters, and especially over the haunches (Fig. 16–1). More general lesions include induration, acute inflammation, central ulceration, circular crusting lesions with either collarettes or peeling peripheral margins, and seborrhea. Pruritus of varying intensity is a constant finding. Obviously, then, lesions of bacterial sensitivity are not much different from those of any other allergy, so the clinician must develop a "sense" of the problem, to begin suspecting and diagnosing bacterial sensitivity.

Diagnosis

Biopsy and histopathology may suggest an immune reaction, but they are not specific in themselves. Therefore, response to antibiotic therapy and intradermal skin testing are the two basic procedures for making a diagnosis, although these measures can also result in an inaccurate diagnosis. If the patient has an underlying locus of infection, lesions and pruritus should respond to appropriate antibiotics. I have had an impression, however, that some antibiotics, particularly the cephalosporins, have inherent antipruritic properties, and combined with their effect on secondary surface bacteria, they may have misleading results. I prefer to use an intradermal skin test. Even though this test also has its problems with inaccuracies, it generally gives you a presumptive, although not an absolute, diagnosis of staphylococcal allergy within minutes or hours.

My choice of skin-test antigen is Staphoid A-B (Coopers-Pitman Moore), a staphylococcal toxoid. It is diluted with an equal volume of saline, and .02 to .03 ml of the diluted toxoid is injected intradermally. Because of the inherently irritating properties of this toxoid, an initial wheal is almost always present; this wheal may fade in 15 to 30 minutes and does not in itself constitute a positive reaction. Therefore, the test must be read critically, and to be positive, the reaction must persist and perhaps even grow larger. If it does fade, a positive delayed-type reaction may develop in 24 to 72 hours, characterized by induration, erythema, and even cratering or central necrosis of the test site. Therefore, if one sees no persistent immediate reaction, the animal must either be returned for 24-, 48-, and 72-hour readings, or the owner must be instructed to call and report each day on the appearance of the injection site.

Treatment

Unless the patient has an active, concurrent infection, antihistamines and antibiotics are of limited value. Corticosteroids afford some temporary relief, but they often become totally ineffective within a short time.

The treatment of choice is to use staphylococcal toxoid, in gradually increasing doses (Table 16–1). Use an 8-dose series, giving the first 5 doses daily or as close to daily as possible, and the last 3 doses 1 week apart.

The method of administration is important

Table 16–1. Dose Schedule For Staphylococcal Toxoid

Dose No.	Amount (ml)	Dose No.	Amount (ml)
1	0.25	5	1.25
2	0.50	6	1.50
3	0.75	7	1.75
4	1.00	8	2.00

when using toxoids, if maximum response is to be achieved; 0.10 ml of each dose is always administered intradermally, with the balance split between subcutaneous and intramuscular routes. This dose schedule and therapeutic regimen are based on the experimental work of Greenberg and colleagues in which toxoids given subcutaneously to rabbits produced high antibody titers, but were not protective against lethal doses of staphylococci.[1-4] When a small portion was administered intradermally, the rabbits then became resistant to challenge. The investigators erroneously postulated the development of a local tissue immunity, but it is now apparent that the intradermal administration was important in initiating a strong cell-mediated immune response by bringing the antigen into close contact with the dermal Langerhans cells. Staphylococcal toxoid seems to be both a specific and a nonspecific cell-mediated immune stimulant, in that it not only activates lymphocytes against specific staphylococcal antigens, but also may help to stimulate some cases of suppressed T-cell function.

Adjunctive antibiotic therapy may also be of value in treating staphylococcal or other bacterial hypersensitivity, especially in the presence of a low-grade or persistent locus of infection. One should use bactericidal drugs and continue therapy for a minimum of 3 weeks. If clinically evident pyoderma is also present, treatment should be continued for at least 5 weeks; all signs of infection must be gone for at least 10 days before antibiotic administration is stopped. After 5 weeks of treatment, one should probably switch to another class of antibiotic. Clinical evidence suggests that the effectiveness of both toxoid and antibiotics is enhanced by combined therapy. For recommended antibiotics and their dosages, see Table 12–2.

ANAL SAC DISEASE AND THE SKIN

If the readers of this text are representative of the veterinarians I regularly meet at lectures and seminars, probably at least 50% received either minimal or no information in veterinary school about anal sacs, their function, and their diseases. In addition, at least this number, or more, have not removed anal sacs, or they shy away from the surgery when confronted with an anal-sac problem.

My first experience with anal sacs occurred shortly after going into practice. A large, mixed-breed dog was presented with pus pouring from the anal sacs and a chronic perianal dermatitis extending onto the ventral surface of the tail. I do not ever remember hearing the words anal sacs mentioned while in veterinary school, and because these were the presteroid days—actually we were barely into the antibiotic stage—I began symptomatic treatment with hot packs and expression of the sacs. As the condition worsened, and as I realized it was time to institute more specific measures, I summoned a classmate and we proceeded to remove these anatomic structures about which we knew practically nothing. Even my anatomy text mentioned them almost in passing. Four hours and an incalculable amount of blood later, the sacs were out, and miraculously, the dog survived. Of equal importance, the dermatitis cleared, the perianal inflammation disappeared, and the dog's coat began to look and feel much better. At that moment, I knew it was time to learn more about anal sacs, the diseases they produce, and their management.

Anatomic Considerations

Anal sacs, often erroneously called anal glands, are bilateral pyriform structures, roughly the size of a hazelnut, lying under the skin lateral to the anus and between the internal and external anal sphincters. The globular body communicates with the outside through a short neck that opens in the anal fold, usually between the two and four o'clock positions. The blood vessels of surgical importance are the caudal hemorrhoidal, perineal, and caudal gluteal arteries and their respective accompanying veins. During surgical removal of the anal sacs, these vessels must be either carefully stripped from the sac wall by blunt dissection or double ligated and divided. Otherwise, one risks being splattered by an artery spurting under high pressure.

The lining of the anal sac is a silvery, blue-gray with a dull sheen. The fundus of the sac is lined by large, coiled tubules of apocrine sudoriparous glands, whose content empties into the lumen. In addition to the apocrine glands, the duct also contains large sebaceous acini. The wall of the sac, therefore, is the true parenchyma, whereas the lumen is merely a reservoir. Therein lies the problem. Once bacteria that inhabit the sac colonize the glandular structures themselves, medical treatment becomes virtually useless. Although one may instill antibacterial medications into the sacs, it is extremely difficult for these medications to work their way into the glands and destroy the bacteria. Surgery, then, ultimately becomes the only treatment of value.

Function

The anal sacs are not essential to the functional integrity of the body but play an important role in the social interaction among dogs, and probably among cats, as well. Anal sac fluid apparently contains a species-specific scent as well as a scent specific to the individual. This is probably the reason that dogs spend a considerable amount of time at anal sniffing when introduced to each other for the first time, spending progressively less time at anal sniffing at each subsequent encounter. Finally, they give no more than a cursory sniff, and off they go.

Teleologically, they may have been developed originally as an offensive or defensive weapon, as well as an identification. When observing frightened dogs on the examining table about to take flight, it is not unusual to seen them lift their tails and express a few drops of anal sac fluid as they attempt to leave the table.

Clinical Signs

The most common clinical sign is "scooting," sitting on the haunches and dragging the anus along the floor or a roughened surface. Other signs of irritation include backing

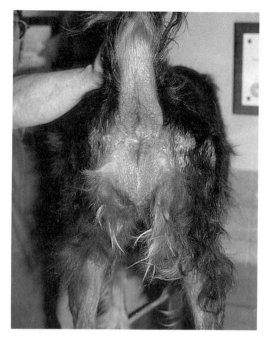

Fig. 16–2.   Dermatitis in a dog with anal sac infection.

up against any rough surface and rubbing the anus and chewing or licking the perianal area, the tail head, and the gluteal region. Clinical signs are not always seen, however, and occasional dogs and cats with severely infected anal sacs have none of these signs. Allergic and other dermatologic signs are often associated with acute, subacute, and chronic anal-sac infections (Figs. 16–2 and 16–3).

The character of the anal-sac content is also a clue, and any dog or cat presented for routine physical examination, vague pain or discomfort around the hindquarters, or a dermatologic condition, must have a rectal ex-

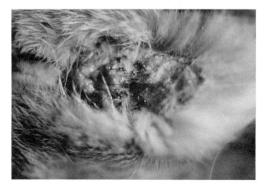

Fig. 16–3.   Perianal inflammation caused by infected anal sacs in a cat.

amination and anal-sac evaluation as part of the examination. The sacs can be expressed and the content examined by placing a tissue or cotton wad over the anus, then grasping the sacs on either side and gently squeezing. No substitute exists for the gloved finger, however, because one may then evaluate not only the content, but also the size, shape, and character of the sacs. To detect apocrine gland tumors of the sacs, for example, is almost impossible without proper rectal palpation.

The anal-sac fluid is normally fetid, watery, and light brown, often flecked with solid brown particles. The infected content ranges in character from dark brown and pasty to creamy, purulent yellow, green, and even hemorrhagic.

Anal Sac Infection

Nonallergic clinical signs associated with infection include bulging of the sac area, cellulitis and inflammation of the skin and subcutaneous tissues overlying the affected sac, pain, and rupture of the sac content through the skin (abscess). Following discharge of the infected content, healing usually occurs spontaneously within a few days, only to recur within weeks, months, or even years.

Treatment consists of administering systemic antibiotics, flushing the sac through its orifice, instilling an antibacterial preparation into the fundus, giving sitz baths, and applying hot packs. If the anal sac has ruptured, it should still be flushed, to drain all infected material through the abscessed opening. Because of the invariable tendency for sacs to reinfect and again abscess at some future date, the ultimate treatment recommendation is total surgical removal. It is not enough to remove just the infected sac; the contralateral sac should be removed as well because later infection of the other sac is common. Because of the amount of inflammatory reaction surrounding the healing abscess, one should wait at least a month after infection before performing the operation, to allow time for the affected tissue to consolidate and contract.

Anal-Sac-Associated Allergic Dermatitis

Allergic dermatitis associated with anal-sac infections is not distinguishable from any other allergic dermatitis, regardless of cause. The first clue, therefore, to the involvement of the anal sacs in a specific clinical problem is the presence of nonspecific clinical signs, particularly scooting, generally associated with irritation, impaction, or infection of the sacs.

Skin lesions are usually located around the hindquarters, especially over the tail head, lateral thighs, and flanks, although they can be found anywhere on the body. Typically, they start as small, pruritic, alopecic, exudative patches that spread or coalesce. Seborrhea is common, and dander and scale may be scattered throughout a dull and lifeless coat. Pruritus also may be localized or widespread.

The diagnosis is presumptive until the anal sacs are removed; that is, anal-sac disease may be suspected based on location of lesions, character of anal-sac content, and behavior typical of anal-sac disease, but a final diagnosis depends on the condition clearing permanently following anal-sac removal. If the condition improves after the sacs are expressed and an antibacterial preparation is instilled, one will have every reason to believe the presumptive diagnosis is accurate. Failure of the condition to improve following medical therapy does not mean a mistaken diagnosis, however, because the infection may be too deep seated, or other unknown factors may be involved, such as concurrent inhalant or food allergy. In general, infected anal sacs coupled with skin disease, particularly involving the posterior third of the body, are a sufficient indication for surgical removal.

Treatment

The treatment of anal-sac-associated allergy is the same as that of anal-sac disease. It consists of emptying the sacs and instilling an antibacterial preparation initially, followed by surgical removal of the sacs. The most important thing to remember about the operation is that the entire sac, including the neck and orifice, must be removed if surgery is to be effective. Surgical texts may contain instructions to isolate the neck and amputate it at the stump, but if any part of the neck and orifice, or any other part of the sac, for

that matter, is left in the body, the problem will most probably return. I have seen innumerable patients with anal-sac allergy improve soon after surgery, only to begin relapsing several weeks later. In each case, the orifice and small secreting portions of the neck (usually less than 2 mm) had been left. Cauterization of the tissue usually fails, and surgical removal of the remaining tissue is the only effective treatment. One other word of caution: cryosurgery should not be used in removing anal sacs because these procedures generally are disasters, either because fistulae are created or because the orifice is sealed off, leaving secreting tissue under the skin.

Preoperative preparation in the same as for any perianal surgical procedure. A complete blood count, serum chemistries, and urinalysis are performed, the patient is fasted overnight, and water is withheld after midnight. An enema on the day of surgery is essential, and it is desirable to administer one on the day before, as well. The entire perianal area is shaved, washed with an antibacterial cleansing preparation, and painted with a nonirritating antiseptic solution, such as povidone-iodine or chlorhexidine.

The sacs should then be emptied, and a suitable packing material injected into them through the orifice. After experimenting with a variety of preparations, I have found Kerr's Syringe Elasticon, a silicone latex emulsion available from any dental supplier, best suited to my needs. A glob of the emulsion is mixed with a few drops of activator (Fig. 16–4), and while the material is still fluid, it is instilled into the sacs (Fig. 16–5). Special equipment is available for this procedure, but merely packing the emulsion into a curved-tip plastic syringe (Fig. 16–6), such as is available from Monoject, works just as well. A pursestring suture may be placed in the anus, if desired, but be careful not to occlude the openings to the sacs. The emulsion cures to a firm, rubbery consistency within about 5 minutes, during which time surgical preparation can be completed.

Positioning of the animal is extremely important and can make the difference between an open, exposed surgical area and one that is obstructed. Most descriptions call for plac-

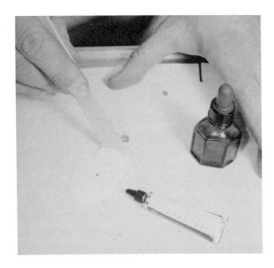

Fig. 16–4. Silicone/latex emulsion and activator used for packing anal sacs prior to surgery.

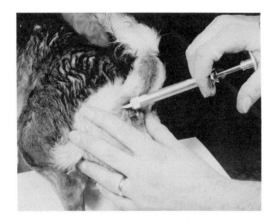

Fig. 16–5. Packing the anal sacs.

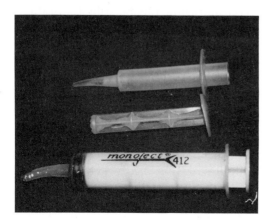

Fig. 16–6. Plastic, curved-tipped syringe suitable for instilling antibacterial ointments into the anal sacs.

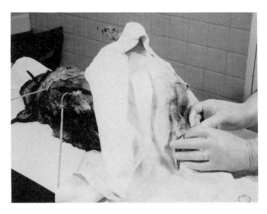

Fig. 16–7. Recommended positioning for surgery. Front feet are tied toward the rear and the hind feet are drawn forward. Tail drops out of the way and perineum can be elevated to any height by drawing hind feet forward.

ing the patient in ventral recumbency and tying the tail forward, over the back. With this technique, it is difficult to position the tail directly over the back without its falling or shifting to one side, thereby occluding the surgical area.

Instead, the patient should be placed in dorsal recumbency (Fig. 16–7), using sand bags if necessary, to keep the animal vertical. With the dog or cat on its back, its hind legs should be drawn forward and tied, while its fore legs are pulled and tied to the rear. By applying tension to the tapes on the hind legs, one can elevate the pelvis to the desired height and the surgical table can be tilted to an angle suitable to the surgeon; the patient's tail just drops conveniently out of the way. Exposure is excellent even in animals with short, stubby tails (Fig. 16–8).

Grasping the anal sac between the thumb

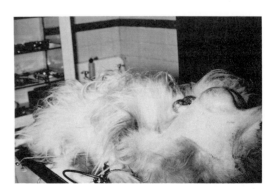

Fig. 16–8. Bilateral perineal hernias exposed for surgery using anal sac tie-down technique.

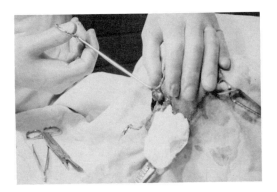

Fig. 16–9. Exposed intact anal sac containing silicone/latex emulsion, dissected free.

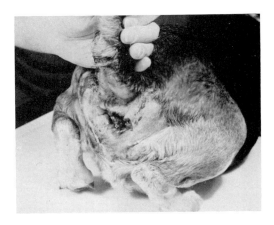

Fig. 16–11. Post-surgical appearance, showing incisions healing by second intention.

and forefinger, make an incision carefully over the fundus, until the sac wall is seen. Using blunt dissection, gently tease the wall away from the surrounding connective tissue stroma; avoid the arterial blood supply, if possible. Bleeding vessels should be ligated immediately to keep the surgical field clear, as well as to prevent retraction into the perineal fat, which makes vessels difficult to find later. Continue dissection along the neck to the orifice, and remove the entire organ intact (Figs. 16–9 and 16–10). **REMEMBER: EVEN THE SMALLEST AMOUNT OF SAC TISSUE LEFT IN SITU WILL ALMOST GUARANTEE A TREATMENT FAILURE.**

Dead space and the skin can be sutured closed, or the entire area can be left open to heal by second intention (Fig. 16–11). Wounds heal equally well using either technique, with but a minor difference in healing time. Cosmetically, results are identical, except for the first few days after surgery. The

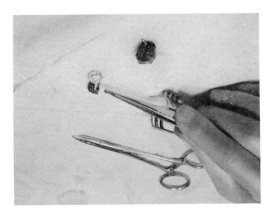

Fig. 16–10. Extirpated sac opened to show solid silicone/latex ball conforming to shape of anal sac.

major disadvantage to open healing is the tendency for drainage during the first few days, but this is offset by the lower incidence of surgical infection. An antibiotic can be given prior to surgery and for several days thereafter.

The principal surgical complication is persistent fecal incontinence in an occasional patient, caused by severing of the anal sphincters. This problem usually resolves as strong fibrous connective tissue fills the area. If not, a row of cautery points can be placed on either side of the anus between two and four o'clock. The resulting inflammation and contraction are usually sufficient to correct the problem.

One should not hesitate to remove the anal sacs because the technique is neither difficult nor complex, surgery can be completed quickly, and results can be gratifying.

One final word: Always remove both sacs; no purpose is served by removing just one. In general, if one sac is infected, the other will probably also be infected, even if to a lesser extent. Anal sacs are time bombs and even if only one sac is infected when the diagnosis is made, the other will probably become infected in the future and will require surgical treatment at a later date. Once the animal has been prepared and positioned for the operation, it take little more effort to remove both anal sacs. Remember, the sacs serve no essential function and there should be no hesitancy about removing them once a problem has developed in either sac.

REFERENCES

1. Greenberg, L., and Cooper, M.Y.: Polyvalent somatic antigen for the prevention of staphylococcal infection. Can. Med. Assoc. J., *83*:143, 1960.
2. Greenberg, L., Cooper, M.Y., and Healy, G.M.: Staph polyvalent somatic antigen vaccine. Part II. An improved method of preparation. Can. Med. Assoc. J., *84*:945, 1961.
3. Greenberg, L., and LeRiche, W.H.: Staphylococcal enzyme lysed soluble vaccine. Med. Serv. J. Can., *17*:581, 1961.
4. Greenberg, L., and LeRiche, W.H.: Staphylococcal enzyme lysed soluble vaccine. Can. J. Public Health, *52*:479, 1961.

Addendum:
Getting Started

We have now come full circle and are finishing where we probably could have started. Just as a journey of a thousand miles must start with the first step, no one will care for and treat allergic pets unless a firm decision is made to start. But how?

First, developing a good basic library is important. It does not have to be extensive, but should contain the information needed to understand problems as they arise. General source materials should include at least one good text on veterinary immunology, a good text on clinical allergy, and at least one good human allergy journal. Also desirable are publications distributed by allergy laboratories and medical institutions.

Excellent basic texts on veterinary immunology are the third edition of Ian Tizard's *Veterinary Immunology: an Introduction* and Halliwell and Gorman's *Veterinary Clinical Immunology,* both published by W.B. Saunders. Also helpful is a good basic human immunology text, such as any current text written by Joseph Bellanti.

Human allergy texts should be available for reference. In this regard, especially for the inexperienced veterinarian, some of the older texts have more basic information. One of the best, in my opinion, is the second edition of *A Manual of Clinical Allergy,* by Sheldon, Lovell, and Mathews. This book is no longer in print, so one can probably find it only in a medical library or used medical book store. Among the newer excellent, but more technical, books are *Allergic Diseases From Infancy to Adulthood,* by Bierman and Pearlman (W. B. Saunders), and *Food Allergy and Intolerance,* by Brostoff and Challacombe (Bailliere Tindall).

Several allergy journals are available; unfortunately, they seem to become more esoteric every year. The *Annals of Allergy,* however, which is the official publication of the American College of Allergy and Immunology, is worth subscribing to because it still contains many excellent clinical papers that are applicable to veterinary practice. In addition, they publish the proceedings of the International Food Allergy Symposia, held periodically since 1972. Subscriptions can be obtained by writing to

The American College of Allergy
and Immunology
800 E. Northwest Highway
Suite 1080
Palatine, IL 60067

The National Jewish Center for Immunology and Respiratory Medicine (1400 Jackson St., Denver, CO 80206) is one of the finest clinical, teaching, and research facilities in the world. In addition to hosting frequent seminars and symposia on all aspects of allergic, respiratory, and immunologic disorders, this center publishes a variety of informative booklets for patients, as well as monthly and quarterly publications describing current research and concepts. These publications, *New Directions* and *Medical Scientific Update,* can be obtained by writing to the public affairs division of the hospital.

Another publication available without charge is the *Pollen and Mold Bulletin,* published weekly from spring through the fall by Nelco Laboratories (see section on allergenic extract suppliers). Although the weekly mold and spore counts are of limited use to most veterinarians because they refer specifically to their location on Long Island, the publication contains information not readily found elsewhere on various mold spores, pollen grains, and the plants from which they come.

Any veterinarian with even a passing interest in allergy should join the Academy of Veterinary Allergy, which conducts an excellent annual scientific meeting, with papers of both clinical and scientific interest, and publishes an informative quarterly newsletter. Applications for membership should be made to the current chairman:

Dr. Richard J. Rossman
330 Waukegan Rd.
Glenview, IL 60025

A final step in the development of a good reference library is the collection of journal articles and reprints. Because no one journal is dedicated to veterinary allergy, reports and articles are scattered among a host of veterinary, medical, and other scientific publications. In addition to filing articles so the information can be easily retrieved, one should review the bibliography, and if the title sounds interesting, write to the author or order it from a medical library. It is amazing how quickly a reference file can be established by an interested veterinarian.

After establishing a library and joining the Academy of Veterinary Allergy, the next thing to do is to become friendly with an allergist interested in either animals or comparative medicine. Before initiating a test-and-treatment program, you should discuss the significant allergens used in his practice. Determine which allergens he considers essential for a basic screening program, as well as those to add for a more extensive program. Allergists can be invaluable resources for veterinarians, to keep them informed of new trends in allergy, day-to-day changes in aeroallergens, diagnostic procedures, and continuing-education programs. Many veterinarians are reluctant to approach physicians initially. Yet any veterinarian who has attended a human allergy association meeting, or who has heard an allergist speak before a veterinary group, soon realizes that most are friendly, helpful people, just as interested in what you are doing as you are in them and their work.

Another invaluable resource for basic, practical information are the sales and technical representatives of the various suppliers of allergenic extracts. These representatives are familiar with the significant allergens present in your practice area and, once your allergy practice is established, can advise you on which allergens to stock and in what concentrations. Companies can also provide you with technical publications, weekly pollen counts, and other valuable services. Companies supplying allergenic extracts to veterinarians are as follows:

Center Laboratories
39 Channel Dr.
Port Washington, NY 11050

Greer Laboratories
PO Box 800
Lanoir, NC 28645

Hollister Stier Co.
400 Morgans Lane
West Haven, CT 06516

Nelco Laboratories
154 Brook Ave.
Deer Park, NY 11729

Finally, virtually every section of the country has regional hospitals that supply regular mold and pollen counts to physicians and other interested people. Such hospitals are good resources during the allergy seasons.

Suggested Readings

Books

Bellanti, J.I.: Immunology. Philadelphia, W.B. Saunders, 1971.

Bierman, C.W., and Pearlman, D.S. (Eds.): Allergic Diseases from Infancy to Childhood. Philadelphia, W.B. Saunders, 1988.

Brostoff, J., and Challacombe, S.J. (Eds.): Food Allergy and Intolerance. London, Bailliere Tindall, 1987.

Douglas, W.W.: Autocoids. *In* Goodman and Gilman's The Pharmacological Basis of Therapeutics, 7th Ed. Edited by A.G. Gilman, et al. New York, Macmillan, 1985.

Halliwell, R.E.W., and Gorman, N.T.: Veterinary Clinical Immunology. Philadelphia, W.B. Saunders, 1989.

Lockey, R.F., and Bukantz, S.C. (Eds.): Principles of Immunology and Allergy. Philadelphia, W.B. Saunders, 1987.

Sheldon, J.M., Lovell, R.G., and Mathews, K.P. (Eds.): A Manual of Clinical Allergy, 2nd Ed. Philadelphia, W.B. Saunders, 1967.

Tizard, I.: Veterinary Immunology: An Introduction, 3rd Ed. Philadelphia, W.B. Saunders, 1987.

Journals and Journal Articles

Annals of Allergy: Part II: Second International Symposium on Immunological and Clinical Problems of Food Allergy. Milan, 1982.

Annals of Allergy: Part II: Food Allergies and Intolerances: A Nestle Foundation Workshop, Lausanne, 1983.

Annals of Allergy: Part II: Sixth International Food Allergy Symposium, Boston, 1987.

Baker, E.: Staphylococcal disease. Vet. Clin. North Am. (Allergy), *4*:107, 1974.

Baker, E.: Allergy skin testing in the dog. J. Am. Vet. Med. Assoc., *148*:1160, 1966.

Baker, E.: Diseases and therapy of the anal sacs of the dog. J. Am. Vet. Med. Assoc., *141*:1347, 1962.

Barr, S.O.: Allergy to Hymenoptera stings: review of the world literature 1953–1970. Ann. Allergy, *29*:49, 1971.

Bernton, H.S., McMahon, T.F., and Brown, H.: Cockroach asthma. Br. J. Dis. Chest, *66*:61, 1972.

Chamberlain, K.W. (ed.): Vet. Clin. North Am. (Allergy), *4*:1, 1974.

Chamberlain, K.W., and Baker, E.: A brief discussion of allergic diseases of other organs and systems. Vet. Clin. North Am. (Allergy), *4*:175, 1974.

Dillon, A.R., Spano, J.S., and Powers, R.D.: Prednisolone-induced hematologic, biochemical and histologic changes in the dog. J. Am. Anim. Hosp. Assoc., *16*:831, 1980.

Fehrer, S., and Halliwell, R.E.W.: Effectiveness of Avon's Skin-So-Soft as a flea repellent in dogs. J. Am. Anim. Hosp. Assoc., *23*:217, 1987.

Hoffman, D.R.: Allergens in Hymenoptera venom. Ann. Allergy, *40*:171, 1978.

Kessler, F.: Hydroxyzine HCl in the management of allergic conditions. Clin. Med., *74*:37, 1967.

Morrow, M.B., Meyer, G.H., and Prince, H.E.: A summary of airborne mold surveys. Ann. Allergy, *22*:575, 1964.

Pichler, M.E., and Schick, R.O.: Safe and effective flea control. KalKan Forum, *4*:60, 1985.

Pinsker, W., and Thayer, K.H.: Treatment of allergic conditions with methysergide (1-methyl-D-lysergic acid (+) butanolamide bimaleate), a new antiserotonin drug. Ann. Allergy, *21*:200, 1963.

Rajka, G.: Studies in sensitivity to molds and staphylococci in prurigo Besnier (atopic dermatitis). Acta Derm. Venereol. (Stockh.) *43 (Suppl. 54)*:43, 1963.

Rhodes, K.H., Kerdel, F., and Soter, N.A.: Comparative aspects of canine and human atopic dermatitis. Semin. Vet. Med. Surg. (Small Anim.), *2*:166, 1987.

Rhodes, K.H., et al.: Investigation into the immunopathogenesis of canine atopy. Semin. Vet. Med. Surg. (Small Anim.), *2*:199, 1987.

Scherago, M., Berkowitz, B., and Reitman, M.: Standardization of dust extracts. Ann. Allergy, *8*:437, 1950.

Scott, D.W., and Buerger, R.G.: Nonsteroidal anti-inflammatory agents in the management of canine pruritus. J. Am. Anim. Hosp. Assoc., *24*:425, 1988.

White, S.D., and Ohman, J.L.: Response to intradermal skin testing with four cat allergen preparations in healthy and allergic dogs. Am. J. Vet. Res., *49*:1873, 1988.

Yanni, J.M., Halliwell, R.E.W., and Tracy, C.H.: Effect of AHR-5333 on flea antigen extract-induced skin reactions in flea-allergic dogs. J. Vet. Pharmacol. Ther., *11*:221, 1988.

Index

Page numbers in italics refer to figures. Page numbers followed by a "t" refer to tables.